Devil's Claw Root
and other natural remedies for
arthritis

Devil's Claw Root
and other natural remedies for
arthritis

Updated and Revised by **Klaus Kaufmann**

Rachel Carston

Published by Alive Books
7436 Fraser Park Drive, Burnaby, BC V5J 5B9

Cover design: Bill Stockmann
Design & typesetting: Sheila Adams & Janet Septhon

First Edition:
    First printing May, 1978
Second Edition:
    First printing: January, 1980
    Second printing: January, 1985
Third Edition:
    First printing April 1994

Canadian Cataloguing in Publication Data
Carston, Rachel.
    Devil's claw root and other natural remedies for arthritis

    Includes bibliographical references and index.
    ISBN 0-920470-36-X

    1. Arthritis—Alternative treatment—Popular works. 2. Herbs—Therapeutic use—Popular works. 3. Arthritis—Diet therapy—Popular works. 4. Holistic medicine—popular works. I. Kaufmann, Klaus, 1942-. II. Title.
    RC933.C37 1994   616.7'220682   C94-910296-2

Printed and bound in Canada.

Contents

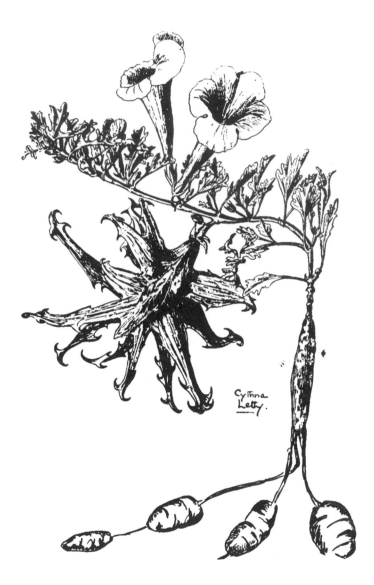

Preface

This revised edition of Devil's Claw Root and Other Natural Remedies for Arthritis comes in response to popular demand. It has been updated and revised to reflect current research and experience with natural treatments for arthritis. Klaus Kaufmann particularly emphasises diet, live foods, nutrients, fasting and rejuvenating therapies.

Natural therapies are becoming more and more accepted in North America. Since the 1980 edition of this book, more information on the relationship between diet and arthritis has become available.

Certain types of food appear to aggravate the condition. Many people have found relief through detoxification and fasting. Identifying food allergies and avoiding allergenic foods has often reversed symptoms. The herb, devil's claw root, has become firmly established as an important component of treatment.

The original author of this work, Rachel Carston, passed away in 1983. Updating was needed before the work could be reprinted. Klaus Kaufmann, author of *The Joy of Juice Fasting*, *Silica – The Forgotten Nutrient*, *Silica – The Amazing Gel*, and *Eliminating Poison in Your Mouth*, fortunately agreed to undertake the needed revisions. He has reworked the text adding to it from his own wealth of knowledge and experience. Opinions and anecdotes expressed in the first person are his.

All of the original information on the causes of arthritis, the different types of arthritis, natural therapies and studies on the effectiveness of devil's claw has been preserved.

Klaus Kaufmann has added sections on anti-allergy diet, alkaline diet, healing by nutrients, detoxification, fasting, massage therapy, cryotherapy and magnetic therapies. He also reports on a new study of devil's claw conducted for the Canadian government's Health Protection Branch. The study clearly confirms the non-toxicity of devil's claw root.

– *Ed.*

> "*But never met this fellow,*
> *Attended or alone,*
> *Without a tighter breathing,*
> *And zero at the bone.*"

Emily Dickinson (1890 AD)

Introduction

The old adage says, "Nature knows best." But does Mother Nature always know best? It seems that, at least in the case of arthritis, the adage is not quite true. Arthritis is a natural, but ultimately incorrect, cellular response to certain stresses on the body. What may be needed then, is an adaptation program to steer the body toward healthy responses without causing unwanted side effects. There is convincing evidence that a herbal preparation called devil's claw root 410 is such an "adaptogen."

In the sixties reports about the health devil's claw root were emanating from England and Germany. Serious scientific studies and hundreds of personal testimonials indicated that this natural organic compound can not only alleviate, but also, in many cases, completely eliminate joint swelling, stiffness and arthritic pain. It seemed too much to hope for at the time.

The root, in concentrated tablet form, has been available in health food stores in the USA, Canada and some places in Mexico, for thirty years. Remarkably it is now sought after by arthritic sufferers more than ever. Such success seems to substantiate the original claims of natural and safe relief from the agony and crippling of arthritis. However, there is still much skepticism from the orthodox medical profession, even in the face of overwhelming evidence collected over the decades by users. While the Arthritis Society still promotes aspirin as a treatment, it consistently ignores other options such as diet, fasting and herbs.

Other health practitioners, frustrated by the drawbacks of pharmaceutical drugs, treat the causes and symptoms of illness differently. Following the tenets of wholistic healing, they view the individual as an integration of mind, body and spirit constantly adapting to the environment. The wholistic approach maintains that arthritis, like most diseases, occurs when the trinity of body, mind and spirit is out of balance. It is well recognized that any successful treatment must proceed wholistically and concentrate on equal treatment of these three pillars of health. Such a treatment provides exercise and diet for the body, stress control for the mind, and a positive attitude and belief for the spirit.

You will read about all of these, including the tools that enable the body to repair itself. With the assistance of diet, nutritional supplements, juices, herbs, exercise to reduce emotional tension and relieve stress, and what might be called a more relaxed, outward looking attitude, the symptoms of diseases seem to disappear. Not because they were miraculously cured overnight, but because, as America's foremost health authority, Dr. Paavo Airola contends, "there would be no reason for their existence."

What does conventional medicine identify as the cause of arthritis, a disease that afflicts three times more women than men? Your doctor, if you are lucky enough to have one who talks your problems over with you, might have mentioned viral infection, auto-immunity, and so forth. Such theories seem, on the face of it, to be completely opposed to the wholistic approach. In fact, a wholistic viewpoint sees the intruding microbe as a *symptom* of the real cause. Wholistic healing searches for the underlying causes, while orthodox treatment looks at symptoms and the treatment of symptoms.

Which of the two comes closest to real understanding, and ultimately to lasting relief of arthritis, is up to you to decide. Arthritis is as complex as it is multi-faceted. It is also highly individual. Each arthritis patient will feel a different set of aches and pains, stemming from causes that particularly affect the individual and may not at all affect their neighbor, friend or relative. Like the cause, the progress of arthritis is totally individual and is often frustratingly unpredictable.

The word arthritis comes from the Greek *arthro* for joint and *itis* denoting inflammation. Conventional medicine uses this word to describe any sign of pain, stiffness or inflammation of the joints. It gives scant attention to the most unique characteristic of this universal malady. no two people ever have identical patterns or progression of symptoms!

Orthodox medicine continues to search for one specific cause (usually a virus or a bacterium) to what is essentially a non-specific response of the body to some form of irritation. After so many years of intensive scientific research, that causative microbe remains as elusive as ever. Could it be that there never was one?

Nutrition-oriented doctors and modern wholistic scientists see arthritis in a much larger perspective. Those are welcome hinges known as joints are, they contend, vulnerable points where any weakness occurring in the system will first reveal itself. In other words, pain and inflammation are the body's way of saying, "Hey, there's something wrong here." The symptoms of arthritis are viewed as signals for help. These signals also indicate that the body is attempting to repair itself and regain its balance. This all-important balance or equilibrium of the body is known as "homeostasis." The ongoing and probably long-standing systemic disturbance can be corrected as the proponents of wholistic healing point out, by aiding the repair mechanisms that are already at work. Thousands of practitioners and previous sufferers around the world agree.

The leading pioneer in this field in America, Dr. Paavo Airola, explains the reasons behind the wholistic treatment of arthritis: "The basic premise is that most diseases have the same basic underlying causes. These are: the systemic derangement and biochemical and metabolic disorder brought about by prolonged physical and mental stresses to which the patient has been subjected – such as faulty nutritional patterns, constant overeating, overindulgence in proteins and the body's inability to properly digest them, nutritional deficiencies, sluggish metabolism and consequent retention of toxic metabolic wastes, poisons from polluted food, water, air and environment, toxic drugs, tobacco and alcohol, lack of sufficient exercise, rest and relaxation, severe emotional stresses, etc."

As stated previously, no two bodies will ever react in exactly the same way. What to your body might be severe stress, can be easily overcome by another. The complete individuality of each of us cannot be overemphasized. Since there are no two identical reactions – or environments for that matter – how can there be identical patterns of joint inflammation and pain? We know there are not. Yet conventional medical opinion insists on the search for one, and only one attacker.

"These health-destroying environmental factors," as we know from Dr. Airola's work, "bring about derangement in all body functions with the consequent biochemical imbalance in the tissues, auto-toxemia (self-poisoning), chronic under supply of oxygen to the cells, poor digestion and ineffective assimilation of nutrients... and gradually lowered resistance to disease. Thus the biological medicine considers not the bacteria, but the weakened organism or the lowered resistance as the primary cause of disease. Bacteria is more often than not, the result of disease, not its cause." [1]

1

The Causes of Arthritis

Orthodox medical science believes that the cause of arthritis is unknown and that the disease is incurable. It reduces therapy to pain-killing treatment. The arthritic is left to look forward to slow and painful crippling. By contrast, more modern research proves that arthritis is essentially a degenerative disease. As such it can be prevented through wholistic approaches and it can definitely be healed in the early stages, and with some persistence and dedication in the later or advanced stages.

Medical textbooks, and as a result, most doctors, distinguish between two types of arthritis; that of the joint lining and tissue – rheumatoid arthritis, and that of the bone – osteoarthritis. The latter, they suggest, is merely the inevitable wearing away of the bone with age. As yet, scholarly medicine confirms that nothing permanent can be done to halt aging. However the study of gerontology often called geriatrics when concerning human aging, is becoming increasingly exciting. Rejuvenation is no longer just the vain quest for the fountain of youth. Living tissue revitalization is a real prospect on the not so distant horizon, and for this reason, deserves its own chapter (see Chapter 7 –

Rejuvenation Can Conquer Arthritis).

Medical research on arthritis is still focused mainly on the rheumatoid form of the disease which, many contend, is not necessarily age-related. Its occurrence in young children confirms this view. We will begin by looking at some of the possible causes of rheumatoid arthritis and will return to osteoarthritis and rejuvenation theories later on.

Persistent Infection

In rheumatoid arthritis, joint tissue inflammation occurs and antibodies are produced as a result. Inflammation and antibodies happen whenever the body mobilizes its defenses to fight off any foreign or toxic invader. For instance, if you cut your finger and the wound becomes infected, the protective response will be inflammation and antibodies. The similarity of the sequence: intervention, inflammation, antibodies – has led some researchers to view arthritis as the result of a chronic viral or bacterial infection.

A number of known harmful organisms experimentally injected into animals can reproduce symptoms which are similar in many respects to arthritis. By the same token, soreness, redness and restricted movement of the joint often erupt in the body as a delayed reaction to an earlier infectious disease such as tuberculosis or venereal disease.

The offending microbe theory, although it still remains pure conjecture, has given birth to some painful and ineffective treatments. You may know someone who had their tonsils removed, or all their teeth pulled, in hopes of thereby getting rid of their sore joints. This latter barbaric treatment was still in vogue a few decades ago when incisors and molars were seen as the breeding ground for infection. It may still be practiced in some medical circles.

How does an infection from the teeth, or wherever, get into the elbow, wrist or knee? Apparently, when arthritis occurs, the structure of the connective tissue of the joint lining (synovium) is altered. Connective tissue was once considered as nothing more than what held the body together. Our living cement it certainly is, but now researchers have found it is also a relatively permeable substance that allows nutrients carried by the bloodstream to pass into the cells, and toxins to exit.

The connective tissue of the synovium, cartilage and bone is composed largely of collagen, an albuminoid material resembling egg white. In arthritis, it has been demonstrated, the collagen weakens and lets fluid and large microbes through into the area surrounding the joint. It is these foreign elements, say the medical scientists, which create the typical symptoms of swelling and inflammation.

The controversy over which comes first – weakened collagen or infectious microbe – is a hot issue in medical journals. Yet rarely is mention made of the proven fact that collagen can be strengthened by diet and vitamin and mineral supplements, particularly vitamins C and D and, latest research indicates, silica. Chapter 5, Live Foods Alleviate Arthritis, will tell you more about this.

While ongoing infection is a very possible and logical cause of arthritis, it is as yet scientifically unclear whether infection is the underlying, or even leading cause of rheumatoid arthritis. There are other possible explanations.

Allergy-Related Arthritis

Arthritics are often predisposed to develop their condition by some fundamental disorder that interferes with the normal process of food assimilation. Gout is one proven example of this. The theory is that an allergy or even a deficiency in a certain nutrient can trigger the arthritic process. However, the main research-funding organization in this country, the Arthritis Society, categorically denies that food intake or diet

3

has anything to do with arthritis. Consequently, research monies to fund the investigation of the relation between food and arthritis are almost non-existent.

The Society contemptuously dismisses the mere mention of diet or allergy as quackery. Yet gout is indisputably a metabolic disorder. It is a malfunction of the body in assimilating purine-containing foods such as meat (liver, sweetbreads), sugar or beer. The critical observer must interject, why not study the possibility of a food connection to other forms of arthritis, which have so many symptoms in common with gout? The food and allergy connection is important. We will look closely at the healing potential of diet in Chapter 5, Live Foods Alleviate Arthritis. Allergies are addressed under the sub-heading Anti-Allergy Diet.

Doctors familiar with nutritional medicine are convinced that the body's reactions to nutrients, including presence of allergy-causing nutrients, imbalance of nutrients and lack of certain nutrients due to deficiency or poor assimilation, all play a vital role in the development and prevention of rheumatoid arthritis. One of the culprits in the more prosperous Western world may be excessive protein consumption (meats, eggs, dairy products). Sustained protein deficiency, almost totally unknown in the West, results eventually in wasting diseases caused by malnutrition. It makes sense then that the reverse condition – excessive protein – may contribute to the cause of arthritis. More abouthat later.

Auto-Immunity

It is a known fact that the arthritic joint lining (synovium) produces antibodies just as a healthy synovium would when resisting a virus. Yet no specific virus has been isolated in arthritis. As a result, another theory is triumphantly produced. "Aha, then the body must be attacking itself!" It is true, such a phenomenon may, at least in part, explain the observed mechanism of synovial tissue and cartilage degeneration. Yet it falls short of pinpointing what starts the process of the body's attack on its joints. What causes some bodies to react with such an obviously foolhardy self-destruction? More questions are raised than answered by this theory.

However, no theoretical problem is insurmountable. To silence any doubts, the two theories are sometimes neatly fitted together. There once was an infectious bacillus, or so the story goes, which completely altered the joint tissue structure. After this, the body no longer recognizing itself, attacked what it saw as a foreign, invading substance. And thus, suggest some researchers, the unnatural battle is joined

Theories Closer to the Bone

Two other hypotheses are tentatively proposed, although they seem to have been as effectively shelved and ignored by the conventional medical experts as the little books in which they are expressed. Arthritis is linked with emotional distress and a certain personality type, concludes Harold Geist, PhD, in his book, Psychological Aspects of Rheumatoid Arthritis. "More recently" he writes, "emotional aspects such as psychic shock and worry have been discovered to contribute to the disease... Rheumatoid arthritic patients were hostile, independent individuals whose ability to express aggression was quite limited. Arthritic symptoms represent a means of controlling or preventing the expression of hostile, aggressive impulses. If the joints are stiff and rigid, motion is limited, anger will be encapsulated and danger to others and oneself will be averted." [2]

In other words, some people are actually aching with hostility and resentment. Such unrelenting tension, frustration or worry eventually drains the body's stress reservoir and lowers resistance and ability to adapt. If the whole mechanism is locked tight and thereby resists release, the eventuality can be drastic. Not surprisingly, it is those human hinges, the joints, that must bear the brunt.

In her book, *Let's Get Well*, Adelle Davis talks of severe and excruciatingly painful arthritis that developed in her jaw and hands when her negative emotions were brought to light. These feelings, experienced in childhood because of her mother's death, had long since been buried in her unconscious. She overcame her arthritic symptoms by expressing her emotions physically. An older female patient of hers also found relief by repeatedly kicking a pillow, thus expelling pent-up hostilities.

In support of this theory, an illuminating sidelight of Dr. Geist's research was the discovery that many arthritics view their bodies as hollow containers – a hard shell with little more than vaporous fluids inside. A perspective of isolation, disassociation and confinement can only be intensified by such a self-image.

Stress

"Rheumatoid arthritis," says Carlton Fredericks, PhD, "is considered by many qualified workers to be a stress disease. Stress is multi-faceted, of course. It can be emotional, or physical. The physical can range from chronic infection, to surgery, to exposure to violently shifting climate." [3]

In a similar vein, Adelle Davis writes, "Studies have revealed that most persons with arthritis have been under severe stress before the onset of the illness; that their diets are appallingly deficient in many respects; and that the level of vitamins in their blood, particularly vitamin C and pantothenic acid, is extremely low... Arthritis remained a mystery until it was shown that remarkable results were obtained when cortisone was given. Obviously, if the body were producing all the cortisone it needed, further cortisone could bring no improvement. Such results indicated that persons with arthritis were in the exhaustion stage of the stress reaction; and that their pituitary and/or adrenal glands could no longer function normally." [4]

These quotations from eminent nutritionists emphasize stress as a cause of arthritis. Does that sound familiar to you? As Dr. Airola explains, the theory of stress is the foundation of "biological medicine." He attributes "lowered resistance to disease" to prolonged physical and mental stress.

Stress is a key word that is much used, but a word whose true meaning many people do not fully understand. People think of stress as a deadline to meet, a fight with their spouse, a flu bug or ptomaine poisoning. Dr. Hans Selye's work on a definition of stress provides a better understanding. Events, called the tensions of living, are stressors. They are the pivots around which hormonal changes occur in the body. Hormonal injections into our blood prepare us for "fight or flight," propel us to action, to survival.

Stress activates a marvelous internal mechanism from the deep well of life within each of us. Whether subconsciously or not, it is understood that this mainspring levers the body into release, physical action, work and creative thought. When denied and suppressed, it runs thwarted like a dammed river, only to undermine its containing banks.

As often as not, it is the mind, and perhaps even what is known as the spirit which perceives an exterior threat and thus initiates the necessary hormonal activity. The mind can choose to view a situation as less stressful or it can imaginatively transform stress into a new and positive energy. If so controlled, the river of life can flow on peacefully, and even power huge turbines.

Definition of Stress

It is unlikely that anyone can find a more complete or authoritative definition of stress than that given by the

Canadian stress doctor Hans Selye, MD:

> "Stress is the state manifested by a specific syndrome, which consists of all the nonspecifically induced changes within a biological system." [5]

In other words, stress is the combination of changes within the body. The changes will invariably occur when triggered by some influence (stressor) which can be almost anything inside or outside the mind-body, hence they are nonspecific.

The stressor is first apprehended by the pituitary gland, a tiny gland at the base of the brain. On being triggered by a stressor, the pituitary produces and sends out the hormones ACTH and STH to initiate protective action by the body. The pituitary's chemical messengers are quickly carried via the bloodstream to the adrenals and stimulate these two small glands (one on top of each kidney) to secrete several other hormones, most notably cortisone.

Cortisone is particularly important in rheumatoid arthritis because it is an anti-inflammatory hormone produced by the body to fight off infection. When directed to an irritated area of the body it will reduce the inflammation that occurred there. As Dr. Selye points out, in cases of really severe dangers, such as tuberculosis, cortisone need not, and indeed should not, be sent out since the inflamed tissue in that instance is preventing the harmful bacteria from spreading to other regions of the body.

With a less dangerous irritant, plant pollen for example, the anti-inflammatory hormone can be safely rushed via the bloodstream to the sinuses. Here, the stimulus is not as dangerous to the tissue as the prolonged inflammation would be.

Just as the mind is often responsible for initiating the appropriate response to a stressor, so the body has to make similar decisions. Is this invading substance antipathetic to the entire organism, or is it simply a mild localized irritant? The body, in a manner of speaking, has to figure out answers to these sorts of questions. Like the mind, sometimes the body makes the wrong choice. When this happens there soon develops what Dr. Selye terms a "disease of adaptation."

"The rheumatic maladies," he explains, "are really typical diseases of adaptation, because if the body's defenses are adequate, the disease is suppressed without any intervention by the physician. Here the primary disease producer (whatever it may be) is certainly not very harmful in itself. When the inflammation barricade against it is removed by hormones, the causative agent (germ, poison) of the rheumatoid diseases does not produce much tissue destruction. These diseases are essentially due to inadequate adaptive reactions against comparatively innocuous injuries. They are due to maladaptation." [6] Just as we can fuss or frustrate ourselves over an imagined slight, so too, can a tissue (in this case the synovial lining) create inflammation to block off what is essentially a slight infection or toxin.

When the swelling, redness and pain around a joint continue, it's a sure sign that the body is not producing or sending enough cortisone to the infected site. Of course, it may not be sending out the hormone because it made the wrong decision, but there are other reasons also. Sometimes, the entire stress response of a living body can get into a groove, a rut. It then needs to be forcibly shocked or lifted into action. (Think of a gramophone needle stuck in an old LP.) This is the reason that such severe stressors as injections of toxic materials or heavy metal preparations (such a gold treatment) can overcome arthritis by jolting the previously inactive glands into production.

Insufficient cortisone production by the adrenals can be directly traced back to poor nutrition. After prolonged stress, the hormones (and their birthplace, the endocrine glands) are exhausted – used up. Nutrients entering the bloodstream are the only raw materials with which they can be replenished and reactivated. The right kind of diet, can naturally and effectively stimulate extra cortisone production (see Chapter 5).

Causes of Osteoarthritis

"Arthritis of the bone" is under a separate heading because medical books usually see it as stemming from causes quite different from those of rheumatoid arthritis. Most often these textbooks view it as an unavoidable ailment of aging, referring to it as a disease of "wear and tear." To those who agree with the wholistic approach to health, that little phrase "wear and tear" is a signal of the possibility that, here as well, the underlying cause is stress. After all, one definition of stress is just that, the "wear and tear" on the body.

In osteoarthritis though, the symptoms can be very dissimilar to those of rheumatoid arthritis. That terrible pain advancing and receding in the joints is still very present, but inflammation does not occur. Rather, the smooth, lubricating ends of the bones (the cartilage) begin to degenerate. Without that natural cushion between parts that are constantly moving against each other, the bone ends begin to splinter and pit. To add to the misery, bony spurs begin to grow, further increasing the pain and restricting mobility.

While the symptoms do not seem to have much in common with hormone exhaustion, Dr. Selye's studies scientifically link this form of arthritis with the stress syndrome. The chemical response here is not hormonal but mineral. In adapting to a stressor, calcium is withdrawn from the bones to elevate the mineral content of the blood. It was found that if the soft tissues are harmed in any way, calcium is laid down in the damaged area rather than returned to the bones. This may explain the high incidence of osteoarthritis among competitive athletes and manual laborers continuously doing very heavy physical work. The physical shock to joints, which prolonged exhausting activities entail, encourage calcium deposits to form around the cartilage. This is certainly one theory that doesn't bode well for joggers.

On the other hand, if osteoarthritis is only an inevitable part of aging and nothing can be done to prevent it, as most mainstream physicians maintain, who can account for the lively octogenarians you sometimes meet? Are they abnormal? Wholistic health authorities argue, they are rather the standard of what life can be like if we follow a preventive approach involving optimum nutrition, herbs, exercise and peace of mind. Before we take a closer look at these aspects of a healthy lifestyle, let us review the common forms of arthritis. Statistics indicate that certain segments of the population are more likely to be affected by one type than another.

2

Different Types of Arthritis

What is this malady that settles in the bones and joints with such agonizing pain? Under the catch-all term of arthritis are listed close to a hundred ailments, each displaying different symptoms. The early stages for them all are similar to what you might feel if you catch a flu bug – a generalized aching throughout the body. What leads doctors to suspect a systemic disturbance as the root cause of these nonspecific pains is the low grade temperature that often accompanies them.

Most noticeable on rising in the mornings, a stiffness begins to hamper the normal movement of muscles and joints. As the disease progresses, the joints become visibly swollen, sometimes red, and any attempt to straighten or bend them brings searing pain. The swellings are often distinctively symmetrical. For instance, if the end joint on the third finger of your right hand is inflamed, you'll probably have the same condition in the corresponding part of the left hand.

Interestingly, the redness and swelling so characteristic of arthritis will usually begin in the digits (fingers and toes), the extremities furthest from the heart. This suggests to some researchers that faulty circulation is involved. Then again, it may be that the body, in its ongoing effort to protect the vital organs, deposits toxic material as far away from the centre as possible, using the extremities as its toxic dump site. This speaks urgently in support of total body cleansing to expel toxins from the overburdened system. Turn to Chapter 5 to find out how to help detoxify your body through diet and fasting.

The very nature of arthritis is so phantasmagorical and at the same time so hellishly real, that giving any more than vague, broad outlines of its initial symptoms is impossible. Pain, stiffness, inflammation – they all come and go, many say without any rhyme or reason. From these early warning signals, the elusive and complex beast can assume many hideous shapes and even become crippling.

Rheumatoid Arthritis

This disease is three times more prevalent among women than men. Such an overwhelming statistic leads a few medical experts to the conclusion that the sex hormones are the culprits medical therapy should be chasing. Yet the malady occurs most frequently in post-menopausal women when hormone levels are low. Thinking back to Adelle Davis and her patient, could the disproportionate number of women be explained by cultural conditioning? Females are often taught to bottle up their hostile emotions while simultaneously discouraged from finding any release through aggressive work, sports or hobbies.

But, health – or the lack of it – is not that simple. All ages and both genders prove susceptible. One out of every fifty in the adult population is afflicted with this form of the disease. It primarily affects the body's connective tissue surrounding the joints. The collagen (cement part of the connective tissue) is probably ruptured or disabled in some way, allowing toxins to attack the joint lining (synovium) which becomes swollen and inflamed. Eventually inflammation spreads over the joint surfaces. The hinges of the fingers, wrists, knees and base of the toes are prime targets.

Osteoarthritis

It is said that everyone will eventually get osteoarthritis if they live long enough. Sounds hopeless, doesn't it? Worse, existing statistics dishearteningly concur with this view. Osteoarthritis is found among the majority of middle-aged and older folk.[7] What can you expect, argue the biological medicine proponents, when we insist on unwittingly insulting our bodies year after year? Is there light at the end of the tunnel?

The accelerated breakdown and disrepair of cartilage and of the other soft tissues (capsule, synovial membrane) – which normally enable a joint to move freely – are what is behind osteoarthritis. There is little or no inflammation. The lack of this symptom (for those who enjoy semantic side tracks) makes the "itis" ending a misnomer in this case. The correct term, which is gaining popularity, is osteoarthrosis.

The weight-bearing stress points like the knee, hip, ankle, back and, notably, the "worked to the bone" fingers are most often affected. Where the cartilage was, small, bony knobs called osteophytes appear. Usually they form only on one side of the bone end, thus interfering with the normal alignment of the joint. The characteristic bend of arthritic fingers is a noticeable result. The key substance in this entire ailment is, of course, cartilage.

The surfaces at the ends of all your bones are slippery, to ease motion. This is due to the cartilage grown there. Seen under a microscope, cartilage is not quite smooth but is pocketed with minute undulations. These tiny folds trap fluid between the two moving parts of a joint. Car owners might expect this lubricant to be a kind of oil. In fact, it is a far more complex and very ingenious watery solution made up of minerals and mucinous protein.

Under pressure, such as when you jump or walk, the joint fluid sheds some of its watery content and thereby thickens. Shock and friction from motion are thus very efficiently and minimized. When the activating pressure, say in your knee joint, is relieved by sitting down, the joint fluid reabsorbs the water and resumes its normal thickness. This thickness is its resting state or state of readiness for impact. When your joint cartilage degenerates, you lose more than lubrication, you must do without the very stuff you can run on. It's not so much like a car without oil as one that can't even get started because the gears are stripped.

Why does the cartilage give out? There are various theories. One is that there is an intrinsic failure of the lubrication process. A second theory says that abrasion outpaces renewal of soft tissue. Another holds that cartilage gives out as a result of fatigue (wear and tear) due to repeated impact shock. In most cases though, the breakdown is accelerated, say nutrition experts, by the predisposing factors of stress and poor diet.

Gout

While the orthodox medical profession is slow to credit other forms of arthritis with a dietary or metabolic background, the cause of gout is admitted, and demonstrated, to be exactly that. How can gout be included under the general term of arthritis by research organizations when at the same time they disregard, and indeed emphatically deny, a similar etiology for rheumatoid arthritis? Dr. Harold Geist is aware of this anomaly when he writes, "Those who argue that rheumatoid arthritis is solely an infectious disease should remember that many of the clinical features are also exhibited by gouty arthritis which is a metabolic disorder." [8]

Described for centuries as the disease of high living, gout is associated with an overly rich diet: lots of meat, particularly organ meats such as sweetbreads, kidney and liver, sugary foods and beer. All these foods are sources of purines which the body converts to uric acid, the waste created by protein breakdown. When it reaches high levels in the bloodstream this acid will precipitate out, that is, solidify into small, sharp crystals, which, as you would expect, irritate the soft joint tissue. Several European doctors believe that similar crystal-like formations are the cause of rheumatoid arthritis.

The extremely painful attacks, that disappear as quickly as they start, are often localized in the big toe. Traditionally, it is men who need that antique piece of furniture, the "gout stool." A certain family pattern or inherited tendency has been illustrated. Genes though, are probably not so much to blame as are food preferences and eating habits passed from father to son.

Ankylosing Spondylitis
Known by the very descriptive phrase, poker back, this disease generally starts as stiffness and pain in the lower spine. Inflammation begins at the entheses, the sites where the ligaments and tendons join the bones. It can then spread to the vertebrae, fusing them into one unbendable unit. Eye, heart and bowel inflammation may also occur. This again suggests the presence of some sort of toxicity throughout the entire body. Not as rare as you might think, ankylosing spondylitis hits one out of every 250 males – females only one tenth as frequently. Exercise, as I discussed in Chapter 6, has proven effective in both preventing and alleviating total rigidity of the spine.

Systemic Lupus Erythematosus (SLE)
SLE is considered to be a collagen disease. The connective

tissue throughout the body becomes inflamed, affecting not only the joints but the skin and internal organs as well. The first symptoms are a skin rash, usually a butterfly-shaped redness across the face, weight loss, low fever, fatigue, anemia and joint pain. Mainly young women between the ages of twenty and forty are afflicted in this way. The section on vitamins (C, E) and minerals (silica) will be of special interest to sufferers of this disease.

Scleroderma

This, too, is a connective tissue ailment. Scleroderma is characterized by a thickening of the skin, most marked in the hands.

Infectious Arthritis

Upon recovery from an infectious illness such as tuberculosis, pneumonia or venereal disease, inflammation and pain can erupt in the joints of both adults and youngsters alike.

Those Little Aches and Pains

Bursitis, a painful condition of the joints, is an inflammation of a bursa, a small fluid-filled tissue sac that provides a cushion between muscle and bone or between two muscles. Injury or over extension of a joint can irritate this tiny, natural ball bearing. Tennis elbow, for instance, often is caused by a bursa being pulled when over-reaching for a stroke.

Fibrositis has fallen out of medical vogue. It used to be a blanket word for any prolonged, otherwise unexplainable ache or stiffness in the muscles. A preponderance of sufferers in this category exhibit similar personalities – tense, nervous, excitable – or have very poor posture. A relaxing form of exercise or massage can be useful for easing the muscular tightness.

These are the most common forms of arthritis. As chronic conditions, they disable millions of Canadians and Americans. For countless thousands more, the flood of pain that constantly advances and recedes is a relentless torture. Fortunately though, stoic suffering is not the only response available to you. There are ways you can both prevent and alleviate many types of arthritis. Your body's natural defenses will protect you if you will only help and reinforce them with nature's own means to overcome disease.

"Arthritis is a serious ailment. Alert yourself to its signs," advises Carlson Wade in his *Fact Book on Arthritis, Nutrition and Natural Therapy*, "and use whatever nature provides to correct its cause and thereby ease and combat its symptoms." [9]

The Arthritis Warning Signs:

1. Repeated pain and stiffness upon arising.
2. Swelling and redness in one or more joints.
3. Pain and lack of mobility in joints.
4. Cold hands and feet.
5. Rash, low fever, anemia, weight loss.

The recommended natural therapies will be described in the chapters following. Let us begin with what seems to be a particularly effective weapon from nature's own anti-arthritic arsenal – a herb. It is the root of a flowering desert plant that goes by the Latin name *Harpagophytum procumbens* or by the folk name of devil's claw root.

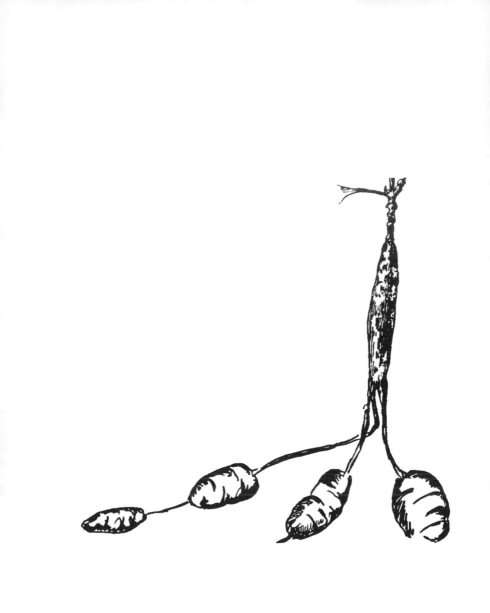

3

The Properties of
Devil's Claw Root

What Is Devil's Claw Root ?

"A renaissance of the remedial plants! Harpagophytum root
provides us with an addition to our armory of medicines
against the poisoning of modern times. It wonderfully stimulates the detoxifying and protective mechanisms of the body"
writes Dr. Siegmund Schmidt in the German journal
Zeitschrift für Naturheilkunde.10 In Namibia (South West
Africa) the great Kalahari desert stretches seemingly forever
in the heat of the day. Extremely dry and practically devoid of
vegetation, it is in this inhospitable terrain, and here alone,
that you will find the marvelous plant Dr. Schmidt was
extolling.

Not so many years ago, a prolonged drought in Namibia all
but extinguished the plant. Only after a drenching, long
downpour did devil's claw happily reappear. The Namibians
were so enthusiastic about this phoenix-like reemergence that
many researchers once again turned their expertise to studying
the plant's medicinal properties. Recent tests have substanti-
ated the local healers' claims for the root of the devil's claw

News of such a natural, harmless remedy could not remain silent for long. Today's naturopaths in Europe and North America recommend the herb. The credit for initially introducing this remedy, and for making the scientific community aware of its anti-arthritic effect, must go to Mr. G.H. Mehnert. He settled in Namibia just after the turn of the century and soon became interested in the herbs and other indigenous vegetation which was so different from anything he had known before. From native savants he learned of their esteem for one particular desert plant. For ailments of the liver, stomach, kidneys, bladder or intestines, they brewed a tea from the dried root of devil's claw. The healing successes, they said, were astoundingly predictable.

But, the traditional use of the herb for relieving the painful symptoms of arthritis, was what Mehnert found most interesting. He devised a way to harvest and prepare the root so that its potency would be preserved even during long storage. Finally, in 1958, he sent samples to Professor Berhard Zorn at the University of Jena in Germany, for him to test devil's claw as a cure for arthritis. Before we look into the results of these experiments, let's take a brief botanical look at *Harpagophytum* and its environs.

Each year, after the first of the Kalahari desert's sporadic but torrential rainfalls, new shoots sprout up from devil's claw rootstocks buried deep in the red, sandy soil. These fragile stems and leaves gradually creep along the ground and eventually produce beautiful red, trumpet-like blooms which mature into thorny seed pods. The pods are heavily barbed and very strong. They can severely injure animals unwary enough to get too close. When local livestock steps on the dried pods, often pliers are needed to pry loose the grip of a pod from the animal's hoof. In fact, the hook-like projections can become so entangled in a sheep's wool that the animal is unable to free itself and must die there. The moisture of the cadaver germinates the seeds. That is indeed a devilish way for any plant to seek its survival. It is due to these pods, which can inflict such damage on the desert tribes' herds that the descriptive folk name evolved.

The devil's claw plant must survive up to ten months of drought a year. It therefore depends on a very deep root system. Along its long root fibers it grows potato-like tubers for storing moisture. In this secondary storage root the medicinal properties of devil's claw are found. The root, when first unearthed, understandably has a very high moisture content. To prevent rot it must be processed soon after harvesting. The water saturation is such that each root provides only a relatively small proportion of active ingredient – six kilograms for every 100 kilograms of tubers.

The tuber is covered with a thin, grooved cork shell. In processing, the root is slit one or two times lengthwise, then slowly dried. As it dehydrates, the strong water-carrying tissue shrinks irregularly to produce characteristic fan-shaped pieces. These are then carefully and painstakingly grated. Mills or knives are not used because the sticky substance would soon coat the metal surfaces and render them useless. So, as you can see, the harvesting of the root is very tricky and time-consuming.

Once grated, it can be brewed as a tea with a very bitter flavor. There is, however, a less bitter form. Tablets pressed from the powdered root, or from a concentrated extract that contains all of the root's medicinal ingredients, are known as devil's claw root 410 tablets. Each of these tablets are equal to 820 milligrams of the original root.

Whom Does It Help ?

In 1976 the teachers and students of St. Joseph's School in England raised money to send their classmate, Karen, a nine-year-old girl to Lourdes. From the age of five, Karen had lived with constant pain and increasing disability. Her father, Colin Brown, in an interview, described the agony she endured. "Karen suffered so much pain that she had to sit on her own so no one would even brush against her." She was given special hospital treatments, everything was tried, but eventually the doctors gave up hope for a remission of symptoms in their young patient.

The trip to Lourdes did not bring any direct relief, but Mrs. Brown now feels that her prayers were answered. Her daughter began herbal treatment in the form of *Harpagophytum* tablets and tea. Within two months, her parents reported that, although it did not completely alleviate the swelling, the herb definitely reduced the pain.

"This is the first time since Karen was struck down with rheumatoid arthritis that she has been able to play like an ordinary child," her grateful mother acknowledged. "Even in the cold and damp weather she is still free from pain." The future looked suddenly bright. Karen had obtained a new lease on life.

George Charles, a 41-year-old father, had given up all hope of leading anything like a normal active life, or of even supporting his family. Ten years of chronic arthritis had completely destroyed all the tissue around his knee and hip joints. Surgery to replace the hip with a plastic counterpart was performed. However, the pain began moving up his body and attacked his shoulders and wrists. Even his work as a salesman, which (with the daily help of 18 pain killing drugs) he was able to do two or three days a week, had to be abandoned. George had to resign himself to a gradually worsening condition, a life of extreme pain and eventual invalidism.

Today, however, he is a new man, working a full week and looking forward to an active future. This virtual resurrection, he claimed, was entirely due to devil's claw root. "I must admit," he says in an interview in the *Liverpool Weekly News*

(November 4, 1976), "that I was very skeptical about the herb. After all, the doctors tried every conventional medicine on me, even steroids, and none of them had any effect. Some days the arthritis would really flare up and I would be unable to move at all. Then a friend told me of a plant called devil's claw which was used in Africa as a panacea and which some German doctors were administering to people suffering from arthritis. Apparently they were achieving exciting cures. I decided that I might as well try it.

"Mind you, I didn't have too much faith in it. But my friend had so much that I thought I may as well humor him. I took the devil's claw root in tea form. And I can tell you that at times our friendship was very strained. The tea was absolutely diabolical to take. It tasted so bitter. But I persevered."

Within five weeks of taking *Harpagophytum*, George was up and about. He even started to fix things around the house and re-tiled the kitchen floor (a job that before the herbal treatment he would never even have contemplated). He found to his great surprise and relief that the swelling in his wrists and fingers receded. He could freely use his hands and shoulders.

"I was amazed," he said. "I can honestly say that I feel like a new man," he added with evident relief. "I no longer have to take so many painkillers. In fact, I only take aspirin in the winter to stave off colds. I feel as if I have been freed. I have a future again."

For the next case history of a 74-year-old, a happy daughter recounts in her own words the relief brought to her formerly bedridden mother. For personal reasons the names must be withheld in this true story.

"My mother has had four weeks' treatment of the devil's claw root, three 410 concentrate tablets a day, and she is going to reduce the dose to two per day for four more weeks. She will then stop taking them. I can't believe the difference. Four weeks ago she was almost speechless and exhausted, nearly out of her mind with the terrible intense pains all over her body. We couldn't leave her bedside as she also felt as if her chest was closing in and almost suffocating her. She just didn't have the strength to breathe. It was heartbreaking to watch.

"She has had a crumbling spine for thirty years, and now the vertebrae which hold the balance of the whole body are disintegrating. The bones press on exposed nerves, causing pain, inflammation and uncontrollable shaking.

"This has now all stopped. She still keeps a box of pain relievers handy in case more pain comes, which it could because of the condition of the bones. But we think that devil's claw root may even heal the bones. It is so marvelous. I just can't find words to describe this wonderful miracle. Even her sight has improved, and she felt hungry after two weeks of the treatment, something she has not felt for years. Before she would eat only a child's meal, having felt so sick with pain. But now she is baking cakes and cooking meals and looking after herself once again."

These three detailed case histories of healing with devil's claw were chosen because of the variety of their circum-stances: a very young girl, an extremely painful condition of a middle-aged father and the rejuvenating miracle of an elderly lady. There are hundreds more. There are many letters and testimonials from people of all ages – each writer grateful and overjoyed with the relief they found in devil's claw root.

The following remarkable testimonial was received on September 1, 1987, from Montreal, Canada:

"I feel compelled to share my recent successful experience with the devil's claw root 410, because I am so grateful. This medication completely healed my rheumatism and arthritis. I am a 47-year-old woman and I have been suffering from rheumatism since I was 18. Pain was my companion for years and I don't count how many physicians... I have seen with no result.

"Lately, I started to have arthritis in my right little finger. So I asked the advice of Gourmand de Nature and was given the devil's claw root extract. After the second day I already felt better, but after one week I had to stop because I underwent gallbladder surgery. After the operation I continued taking the devil's claw medication because my finger ached again and more. I have been taking only this natural medicine for four weeks now and I feel very well. But what is more, the pain in my back and legs (like sciatica) has completely disappeared and I feel like another woman.

"Before, I could not endure a change in weather or humidity in the air. The pain was so awful that I could not stand but had to lie down. I think that the medical profession should know about and prescribe this natural medication. In my opinion, it is the only one able to heal rheumatism and arthritis. With kindest regards, sincerely yours, Benedetta Cherrat.

"P.S.: I also think that the devil's claw helped me recover after the gallbladder surgery. I have seen the surgeon today, five weeks after surgery, and he told me he was very happy with my physical condition and recovery."

Will Devil's Claw Help You?

It helped Karen Brown, George Charles, Benedetta Cherrat and hundreds of others.[11] Arthritis is complex, however. It stems, as we have seen, from what could be any number of stressors and then is frequently complicated by environment, heredity, personality or metabolism. Since the cause is probably never the same for any two people, there are those who find *Harpagophytum* doesn't relieve their symptoms. No one can guarantee that it, or any remedy, will work for you. Yet, as demonstrated in a German study, an average of six out of ten sufferers were able to once again live more fully, more hopefully, because of being treated with devil's claw. Such excellent odds make it worthwhile for anyone suffering from arthritis to try it out for at least one full cycle.

Some medical practitioners may say that the reduction in pain and inflammation is psychosomatic. You think you are going to get better and therefore, you actually do. Others might argue, "Oh, it's just like giving a pink sugar pill – a placebo. The patient at least feels that something is being done about his real or imagined complaint."

No doubt there are elements of hope raised and satisfied by devil's claw root. A wish to get well is of paramount importance in recovery, no matter what the therapy, but a sixty percent remission rate suggests that some very definite physical process is underway here. No matter how much orthodox medicine may pooh-pooh natural healing methods, this herbal treatment does work for many. And that is a standard of efficacy that simply cannot be ignored.

Scientific Studies

For more proof, let us visit with Professor Berhard Zorn, Director of the Physiological and Chemical Institute of the Friedrich Schiller University of Jena. He describes his experiments in the journal, *Zeitschrift für Rheumaforschung*.[12]

"The root of a South West African plant with the botanical name of *Harpagophytum procumbens* DC which belongs to the *Pedaliaceae* family is highly regarded by Africans for its healing powers. It is used in the form of an infusion (tea) in rheumatic disease, diabetes, arteriosclerosis and diseases of the liver, kidneys and bladder. Diseases of the stomach, intestine and abdomen are also apparently benefited. It is said that the complaints of old age are improved by the regular use of the decoction, the hardened vascular walls once again become elastic, and there is a generalized feeling of strength.

"These reports concerning the excellent healing properties of *Harpagophytum* root led us to carry out experimental animal trials. The mode of use, as suggested by Mr. Mehnert, is that of one to two heaped teaspoonfuls of the tea infused (steeped) in about a half liter of water in the evening. This infusion which has an intensely bitter taste, is left to steep overnight, and is then drunk the next day, one-third in the morning, one-third at midday and one-third in the evening.

"As the test model for our investigations, formaldehyde-induced arthritis in white rats was adopted, this having proved best in our earlier investigations of other anti-inflammatory and anti-arthritic compounds. Adult albino rats of both sexes, with an average weight of 175 to 200 grams were used as test animals. The rats were made arthritic in the usual way, by injection in the right hind paw of 0.2cc of a freshly prepared 2 percent solution of formaldehyde. When the joint inflammation had reached its maximum, which was usually twelve to fourteen days later, treatment was begun.

"We were interested to know whether the herb contained an anti-inflammatory or anti-arthritic active principle. Infusions were made and administered both by sub-cutaneous (under the skin) injection and orally via a tube down the throat."

Three series of tests were conducted. In the first group of twenty rats, ten were given daily injections of *Harpagophytum*. The other ten were left untreated and acted as controls. Dr. Zorn and his assistants recorded a pronounced reduction in swelling of the arthritic joints soon after the first injection. The swelling diminished progressively as treatment continued. After about five weeks, the residual swelling was only twenty-two percent of the initial level, and normal movements of the paw were noted.

Meanwhile, the arthritic joints of the control animals remained thickened and showed little spontaneous reduction of swelling. All the injections in this first test were tolerated without irritation, and did not in any way affect the the animals' general health. The most remarkable aspect of the devil's claw root treatment was that even after the injections discontinued "the healing process continued uninterrupted."

In the second test there was an even greater reduction in joint swelling. Extremely large doses were injected in the third test, with fatal results for a few of the test animals. Increased oral dosages produced a rapid and very pronounced anti-arthritic effect, but they were not well tolerated. This series of three tests thoroughly convinced Dr. Zorn of the anti-arthritic and anti-inflammatory properties of *Harpagophytum*. He cautioned that suitable dosage strengths had to be further investigated. Experiments since 1958 have now established safe yet effective levels. The usual nine-week treatment course of the devil's claw tablets corresponds to these guidelines.

"The infusion," Dr. Zorn concludes, "produces a pronounced diminution in swelling with full restoration in joint movement whether administered orally or subcutaneously. It is noteworthy that after treatment has been discontinued, the healing set in motion continues. Lay opinions concerning the healing properties of *Harpagophytum* root in rheumatic diseases can thus be accepted as true and are supported by our animal studies."

You might object that experimental formaldehyde-induced arthritis does not represent a real model of human symptoms and causes. To a certain extent this is true, but an important component of rheumatic joint inflammation is of a nonspecific nature and responds to drugs with anti-inflammatory properties. Scientifically, it has always been accepted that a compound can be called an anti-rheumatic agent if it improves formaldehyde-induced arthritis.

We do not have to rely exclusively on Dr. Zorn to verify African folk wisdom. Since his experiments, several European doctors have treated arthritics with both *Harpagophytum* tea and tablets. Their published reports confirm it as an anti-arthritic in humans. Over five controlled studies on over 350 patients have reported excellent results.

Dr. Siegmund Schmidt of Bad Rothenfelde, Germany, discusses his clinical experience: "I have been prescribing devil's claw root for the past year for my rheumatic patients. It has provided valuable support for the usual rheumatic treatment in more than sixty patients, and for some I have been able to dispense with drugs. In mild cases I have been able to use Harpago tea alone!" [13]

Since the herb was a personally unknown ingredient, this physician first tried it on himself. "I should emphasize," he explains, "that I did not at first believe in the prompt effect of the herb in previous trials I had read about. It was only after personal use that my doubts concerning its therapeutic effect were set to rest. This is what happened.

For more than a year I have had pain in the left knee when I walked and sometimes even when at rest. X-rays showed slight changes. I first injected *Harpagophytum* into the side of the knee joint, 1ml in each side. The pain disappeared after ten minutes and I could move the knee freely. The pain returned twenty-four hours later and I injected 4ml. I was now pain free for two days. Subsequently I increased the total dose to 6ml. The knee joint was then completely asymptomatic, fully movable, and pain-free." [14]

Encouraged by this success, Dr. Schmidt treated more than sixty out-patients. He reported that thirty six, a significant percentage, were soon pain-free and fully mobile. Twelve had less pain and somewhat improved joint mobility, while twelve experienced no improvement. Acute inflammatory conditions, those which flare up sporadically, responded less well than the more chronic conditions, Dr. Schmidt observed. For several of the sixty patients, prescribed dosages of corticosteroids could be reduced by nearly half.

"Excessively high serum cholesterol and blood urea levels also returned to normal during this treatment," adds this German doctor. Such an unforeseen effect, he suggested, is particularly noteworthy since it demonstrates a normalizing systemic influence produced by the herb. And, as you will remember, gout is caused by high levels of uric acid, a component of blood urea. Could other forms of arthritis be linked to it as well?

Harpagophytum procumbens is a completely natural medicine. It has been used in Africa for centuries, and other than slight nausea, usually caused by complicating factors, no harmful side effects from it have ever been reported. Two German researchers, Tunman and Lux, who decoded part of the chemical composition of the herb, did specific toxicity testing on mice. A good tolerance was demonstrated. A Canadian government study also demonstrated no toxicity (see Chapter 8).

The scientists noted that a mouse would have to drink one quarter of its body weight in *Harpagophytum* tea before the herb was anywhere close to being lethal. In such amounts, even water can be harmful. At the Hygen Institute of Graz in Austria, Professor Mose also tried to pinpoint a toxic reaction to the herb. Results correspond with those of Tunman and Lux. As an interesting sidelight, these tests also indicated an inhibition of tumor growth.

Which chemical or combination of chemicals in the desert root alleviates inflammation is not yet established. Analysis is presently under way in several European laboratories. Some researchers have suggested that the diuretic effect, first noted in the experiments of 1958, is probably fundamental to the anti-inflammatory process.

"*Harpagophytum* has a beneficial intermediary influence," writes Dr. Zorn, "which increases the diuretic effect as a result of the dehydration of the dyscolloidal tissue swelling and inflammation leading to a return to normal of the collagen and the impediment of movement and the pain conditions caused by it." In other words, there is a substance here which reduces the inflammation by extracting superfluous fluid from the joint area. The connective tissue can then function normally and once more act as a barrier against toxins.

Some of the active ingredients in *Harpagophytum* have been isolated. In the prestigious *German Pharmacists' Journal*, the chemists Tunman and Lux published their discovery of three of them: the glucosides harpagosid, harpagid, and procumbin.[15] But no matter how much further laboratory sleuthing takes place, it must be remembered that *Harpagophytum* is effective as an natural substance. Its unique and complex structure is bound by nature in such a way that all its parts work in unison. Such a whole remedy, many therapists reason, is much more beneficial than any one single factor synthesized in a test tube.

In comparing *Harpagophytum* to most of the orthodox remedies prescribed for arthritis sufferers, one wonders how so many members of the medical profession can have the temerity to discount the natural, physiological approach. I will be revealing more modern and even more reassuring devil's claw statistics later, but in between let us take a good look at the track record and known side effects of some of the other "wonder drugs" so often recommended for arthritis by well-meaning physicians who follow the orthodox medical school.

4

Natural Therapy vs Drugs

Is Aspirin the Best Medicine?

"For most people with arthritis, aspirin is the best single medicine," reads the opening statement of a pamphlet distributed by the Arthritis Society of Canada. "Aspirin relieves pain," it continues. Everyone would probably agree that it does. But how many acetylsalicylic acid (ASA) tablets do you need to take before pain is reduced? How groggy and queasy do you feel after such massive amounts?

"It also reduces inflammation." [16] Yes, it does that too. In some instances, aspirin may relieve and even treat the common symptoms of arthritis. Even so, many health experts do not agree that aspirin is the best medicine. Inflammation and pain, they argue, are the body's way of coping with a disorder in the joint lining. ASA may alleviate the recognizable symptoms, but in no way can it treat the root cause which is often, as we have seen, a systemic disturbance or imbalance.

Overcome, remove and prevent the cause, say authorities such as Airola and Adelle Davis. Don't just palliate. It is unfortunate that the main fund-raising group for a disease affecting so many should extol aspirin while at the same time denying a role for diet. Which avenues of research are they likely to support: prevention or drug intervention? Why is it that the best-funded organizations are often deaf to the voice of reason? So many of them are steadfastly marching to the wrong drummer, unwilling to unplug their ears even for a moment to listen to a different tune.

However, let us not misunderstand the role of aspirin. Aspirin definitely has a place in the treatment of arthritis. When pain is particularly intense you need something to deaden it, and thank goodness an effective medication is so easily available and so safe. Or is it?

"Overdoses of aspirin cause ringing in the ears and slight deafness. These symptoms go away when the dosage is reduced. And some people can't or should not take aspirin at all because it upsets their stomachs, or because they are allergic to it, or because they have certain conditions – like peptic ulcers for example – which might be made worse," warns the Arthritis Society pamphlet. Apart from the slightly patronizing tone of the advice, does it objectively tell us the whole story? Where is the scientifically documented evidence on the toxicity of aspirin in dosages of 12 to 18 tablets per day, which are not unusual for many arthritis sufferers?

The *Merck Index*, a respected medical dictionary, has a long and frightening list: average doses, but more commonly large doses, may cause tinnitus, nausea, vomiting, diarrhea, gastro-intestinal bleeding. Large doses may, in addition, cause auditory impairment, vertigo, headache, restlessness, hallucinations, delirium, stupor, coma, convulsions, circulatory collapse, respiratory failure, renal damage and death.

Cortisone and Other Steroids

Prolonged stress can so exhaust the adrenals that they are no longer capable of producing enough hormones to suppress inflammation. In such cases, synthetic cortisone is sometimes administered. Most people are well aware of the common side effects of this artificial replacement: round moon face caused by water retention, indigestion or stomach ulcers, increased hair growth in females. Over a prolonged period it can seriously weaken the bones and muscles.[17]

Recommendation for use of this drug is unusual except in extreme circumstances. Where nothing else seems to work, the corticosteroids do miraculously clear up all the signs of arthritis, almost overnight. Such treatment, however, is only a stopgap measure. It can even aggravate the original cause since the endocrine glands quickly become dependent on the newly introduced chemical. Since the newcomer does all their work for them, the adrenals may lapse deeper into inactivity. It is for this reason that cortisone treatment cannot be discontinued suddenly, but must be gradually lessened, under a doctor's supervision. Only gradual withdrawal gives the adrenals a chance to take up the slack.

The moon face syndrome, it has been demonstrated, can be alleviated with the help of a potassium chloride supplement, which reduces water held in body tissues and lowers blood pressure. A diet low in salt, high in protein (not necessarily from meat) and rich in B vitamins can, according to Adelle Davis, decrease many of the toxic effects of cortisone. There are also several diets that help to stimulate natural hormone secretion, as you'll see in Chapter 5.

Drugs That Produce Actual Remissions

Drugs capable of producing remission of arthritis are generally of two types. Both types were originally used to combat infectious diseases. Gold, not the solid metal but a soluble mineral salt, was first injected into tuberculosis patients. Doctors soon discovered that not only the TB but also the arthritis symptoms disappeared. Since they are pouring a very toxic element into the bloodstream, these injections have some extremely undesirable side effects involving the skin, kidneys and blood. They cannot be administered for lengthy periods of time, and if a rash or sore throat develops, treatment must be stopped immediately. Understandably, gold injections are mainly out of medical favor today.

Chloroquine, originally a malaria drug, also proved beneficial in relieving rheumatoid arthritis. But here again, the side effects lead many to reject the cure as possibly more harmful than the disease. It is interesting to note that devil's claw root was also used in Africa at the turn of the century by Europeans as an anti-malarial. There is speculation that it acts like the drug chloroquine to produce a real remission. Yet the herb a natural substance, totally unadulterated and unsynthesized, does not seem to produce the unwanted side effects of chloroquine.

Immunity Suppressors

The auto-immune theory discussed earlier postulates a malfunction in the body's defense system. A group of drugs developed in cancer research suppresses the natural immune system. These pharmaceuticals block what may be an inappropriate immune response, and when deployed against arthritis, they do reduce inflammation. The body, however, is left virtually unguarded against any other bacterial or viral threats.

Practitioners are treating arthritis patients with an unnecessarily dangerous therapy, while the theory behind use of this therapy is disputed. According to Dr. Charles M. Plotz, a famous rheumatologist, "The concept of auto-immunity in rheumatoid arthritis is open to criticism... my guess is that the disease really is not auto-immune but that some extrinsic factor (from outside the body) is involved." [18]

Surgery and Joint Replacement

The marvels of medical surgery and technology can give you a new smooth, plastic pivoting point to replace your worn down old hip. Sadly for many, such an operation is the only path to some modicum of restored mobility. Replacement of other moving parts has not been as successful as for the hip. But why, nutritionists claim, put yourself through the trauma and stress of surgery? Why let your bones degenerate to such a point? Such serious deterioration, they maintain, can be prevented.

You may be undergoing or have undergone one or more of the conventional treatments just mentioned. If so, then you are probably very conscious of the trauma caused by powerful drugs and/or surgery. You, like so many arthritis sufferers, are probably searching for something that can relieve that throbbing pain without adding more to your misery.

Particularly in North America, it is high time that we look more to remedies that, instead of destroying our very tissue and marrow, work in harmony with the principles of life operating within and around us. It is time to turn to the natural world for answers. After all, as physical beings, we are very much a part of nature's eternal process.

"Nature has not given us any disease for which it has not also provided a remedy," is a famous quote from the 18th century Swiss physician, Paracelsus. Work with nature, not against it, if you wish to truly heal yourself – this is the message from the healers of the past.

Herbal Healing
with Devil's Claw Root Is Natural Therapy

"An addition to our natural armory against poisoning," is how Dr. Siegmund Schmidt describes devil's claw root. After personally testing the herb and then prescribing it to several of his patients, another German physician, Dr. von Korvin-

Krasinski, an authority on Tibetan and east Asian medicine, found the desert root equally effective and potent.

"What is so unusual about *Harpagophytum*," he writes, "is its extraordinary versatility as a therapeutic remedy. It would be misleading just to ascribe to it diuretic properties. What is so remarkable about the plant is that it also strengthens the organs such as the bladder and kidney. The bitter taste is gall-releasing. We may conclude that *Harpagophytum* would provide excellent services in the case of gall and liver afflictions as well as cases of pancreas gland insufficiency." [19]

Dr. Schmidt also discovered that high cholesterol and blood sugar levels were normalized during treatment with *Harpagophytum*. Dr. H. Hoppe, confirms this fortuitous attribute. After administering devil's claw root tea to several diabetic patients at a psychiatric hospital, he concluded that, "this trial of a decoction of *Harpagophytum* confirms that elevated cholesterol and neutral fat levels are reduced, and that a good effect is produced on elevated blood sugar levels... The compound may be used as a preventative measure and as an adjunct to diabetic treatment in older patients with diabetes mellitus with elevated serum fats. I recommend it as a very suitable treatment." [20]

Dr. Vogel, the famous Swiss herbalist, journeyed to Africa specifically to study the devil's claw plant in its natural habitat and to question the people about their customs and traditional uses of the root. He reports in his herbal magazine, "South-West Africans [21] maintain that there is no better remedy for purifying kidneys and liver ailments than devil's claw root tea. They are also convinced that it will dissolve and expel gallstones. If anybody suffers from the latter he should make the effort and put it to the test. The tea is completely harmless and will not cause any side effects. It has a purifying value and will be rewarding anyway.

"The tea will also ease complaints of rheumatism and gout. The natives of the seaport Swakopmund in Namibia (South West Africa) are exposed to those ailments especially during the fall and winter months. What a blessing that this very helpful plant thrives nearby to be used as a most reliable remedy. Everybody states that nothing can be compared to the effectiveness of this tea of the desert. The cleansing and curing done within the body by this tea is proven in urine analysis done while under treatment. Such a test will show an astonishing discharge of uric acid, which is the cause of the ailments just mentioned."

So impressed was this learned man by *Harpagophytum* that he now recommends it for everyone. "At least once a year, even the healthy person should plan a cure for his own benefit, especially during the spring, to cleanse the most important organs, lymph and blood. Since pollution of air, water, and food have become a hazard to our health, we should try to relieve our bodies from that added burden. *Harpagophytum* tea will relieve our body of this dross and toxic waste and help us to enjoy a healthier life." [22]

The herb helped Barbara Cartland, the famous English health writer. In the British magazine *Here's Health*, she relates, "I am taking devil's claw tea myself. I certainly think it has a healing effect over my whole body and takes away, almost immediately, any pain or swelling in the rheumatic joints. I had a friend who was suffering from a very irritating skin condition which would not react to any ointment or lotion. She tried dozens and came to me in desperation. I had read that Africans have an ointment for external sores made by powdering the root of the devil's claw. Because I could not get hold of this I put two of the tablets in water and applied the liquid to the inflamed skin. In the twenty-four hours it had healed and she had no more irritation. It was so extraordinary, she could hardly believe it herself!

"As you know I have always believed that nature has a remedy for every disease and condition of the body. Here is something new; here is something which has been closely guarded from the outside world since the beginning of the century. I think we are extremely fortunate that now devil's claw root is available to everyone who suffers from the distressing and persistent diseases which in many cases do not respond to ordinary doctors' medicine."

Dr. Vogel also notes the Africans' use of powdered roots applied to fresh wounds. "Through experience," he adds, "we know that the intake of vitamin C will support and aid the healing. It is advisable to eat two grapefruits or the equivalent in juice daily during the treatment period with devil's claw root."

Some herbs are known and have been cherished for centuries because of their cleansing properties. They are able to wash out the system, and accelerate the excretion of harmful elements accumulated within the body. In this way they aid and stimulate the body's repair mechanisms. A natural remedy is based on the belief that the human body is fully equipped to rid itself of many ailments (short of bullet wounds and similar emergencies) if it is only given the proper aid: an occasional cleansing and optimum nutritional support.

Most orthodox medicine concentrates on chemically synthesized compounds that are designed to eliminate only one specific complaint. Too often (as we have seen with aspirin and cortisone) these limited treatments tend to short circuit the body's defenses and disrupt its adaptive processes. A natural herbal compound works non-specifically and thereby assists the ailing body in its constant efforts to regain the normal state of health. Due to their effort in concert with nature, and not against it, herbs achieve diffuse, yet essentially interrelated results.

Dr. von Korvin-Krasinski found that devil's claw root not only fulfilled all the requirements for a natural therapy, but it also had a bonus. "Quite apart from these wholly beneficial effects upon the kidney, bladder, gall and other organs," he writes, "there is a general feeling of improved well-being. You could compare it with the good early morning feeling after a brief but deep sleep, accompanied with the noticeable relief that climbing stairs is no longer an effort, and you have an idea of the uplift you feel."[23]

Other herbs that herbalists have found helpful in arthritis are: alfalfa as an anti-inflammatory, burdock root for general pain relief, cayenne because it is stimulating, celery seed and chaparral, which are pain-relieving and anti-rheumatic, kelp, which is nutritive, licorice root, again as an anti-inflammatory, and queen of the meadow, also anti-inflammatory and anti-arthritic. Sarsaparilla root is detoxifying and anti-rheumatic, while white willow bark offers pain relief. Some of these can be used as seasonings. Others combined or alone are ideal for teas. None of them, however, is as well documented as devil's claw root.

5

Live Foods Alleviate Arthritis

Society's Diet

Now, we come to what is probably the most contentious issue surrounding any discussion of arthritis. Can diet and vitamins influence, control, heal or prevent this disease? Many nutritionists treat arthritis by prescribing diets. Medical doctors who, in addition to obtaining their regular medical degree, study nutritional medicine not taught at medical school generally agree. Although dietary therapies can appear different and conflicting in particulars, the basic principles are fundamentally allied: the therapies all cleanse and repair the body.

When you undertake one of these programs, don't forget the all important factor of your individuality. Experts like Dr. Roger Williams and Dr. Abram Hoffer emphasize individuality as the substratum of all illness and hence all treatment. Each of us is unique. As an individual constantly adapting to every kind of influence, each of us reacts in our own distinctive way to our environment, to food, to psychological trauma, to life. No two people are ever alike or can respond in exactly the same way, not even identical twins. Nor, by the same token, are any two cases of arthritis totally alike.

You may have had your discomforts diagnosed as rheumatoid arthritis, and your friend's aches and pains may be called the same thing by the doctor. But do not take it for granted that the two conditions are identical. What helps your friend may do nothing for you. Experiment a little with different diets and while doing so listen to what your body is saying. You will be surprised at all the signals it is constantly transmitting. Then adapt your diet to what your body is telling you.

Nutrition, or the lack of it, is what some researchers call a predisposing factor in disease. By this they mean that a deficient or harmful diet actually plows the ground for a grim harvest. Body cells are renewed constantly. What else could new cells be made of if not raw materials extracted from the foods we take in? The human body is marvelously regenerative, but it does not have the ability to synthesize something from nothing. If our bodies do not have enough or the right kind of building material, what do you suppose happens to new cells? There is absolutely no way they can keep doing what they were originally designed to do for us.

You may experience arthritis as a throbbing pain, or redness, swelling and stiffness in a joint. Yet it is the myriad cells of the bone tissue and lining which are unstable, weak, run down, or even deformed. When in such a dismal state, they are no longer able to carry out their assigned functions. You need to feed those cells properly. Help them to be strongly built in the first place and continually send the correct nutrients to support their maintenance. After all, your body can only be as healthy as its weakest cell.

Of the onset of disease, Dr. Roger Williams, the world renowned biochemist and Nobel prize winner, proposed the motto, "If in doubt, try nutrition first." No matter how much like common sense that sounds, the Canadian Arthritis Society rejects it: "The truth about diet and arthritis" they claim, "may surprise you. It is simply this: there is *no* special diet for arthritis. *No* specific food has anything to do with causing it. And *no* specific diet will cure it. "The fact is, the possibility that some dietary factor either causes or can help control arthritis has been thoroughly and scientifically investigated and disproved."[24]

Let's have a closer look at some of these unequivocal statements. The "dietary factor... has been thoroughly and scientifically investigated and disproved." Dr. Roger Williams disagrees. "Even though attempts to treat arthritis and related troubles by nutritional means have so far been limited and inexpert, the results have been exceptionally promising," he maintains.[25]

How much investigation has happened? All research funded by The Arthritis Society concentrates on the virus theory. If you submitted a proposal to study the link between diet and this disease, no matter how well qualified, they would likely turn you down flat. Investigated and disproved? Neglected and despised would be a more fitting description.

Howard Long, president of the Adelle Davis Foundation in California refutes the Arthritis Society position. "I know many people who don't have arthritis any more. Why? They didn't know diet didn't work. It is clear that drugs and devices don't cure, although they may alleviate. The overwhelming evidence indicates that diet does work. The US Department of Agriculture says that "doing nothing but improving nutrition can reduce those suffering (from arthritis) by half!"[26]

"No specific food has anything to do with causing it," says the Society. But purine foods such as organ meats and beer cause gout. No one knows what the inciting factors for other types of arthritis might be. Dr. Collin H. Dong claims that food allergies are the trigger for the entire degenerative process. He has cured both himself and many patients just by altering diet. He gives many fascinating case histories.[27]

Ignoring the whole question of individuality, the Arthritis Society suggests that all arthritics need only a normal, well-balanced, nourishing diet. To be more specific, they advise a daily menu selected from the four food groups in the following proportion:

1. Two or more cups of milk or milk products.
2. Two servings from the meat group.
3. Four servings of vegetables and fruits.
4. Four servings from the bread and cereal group.

Let's review this "well-balanced diet" in the harsh light of North American supermarkets. When eating from the milk group someone might easily choose processed cheeses, margarine or yogurt and feel they had made a healthy purchase. On reading the labels they would find that the cheese is artificially colored, and liberally laden with chemical preservatives. It bears about as much kinship to natural cheese as the margarine does to butter.

Margarine, because of the way it is processed, is not, according to Airola and others, a nutritious food. In fact it can even be harmful. Margarine is manufactured and hardened in a heat process that destroys the unsaturates. Airola and others suggest people use butter, particularly for cooking. Similarly most supermarket yogurts have artificial colors, flavoring, and a high dose of sugar added. All of these foods are nutritionally compromised and yet they make up a large portion of the dairy section in any supermarket.

During a recent medical seminar a doctor related a story concerning war-related food shortages in his native city of Colorado Springs. At the time, many of his neighbors complained that the local supermarket had completely run out of food. Somewhat concerned, he decided to visit the supermarket. He returned with bags full of groceries.

He had found only fresh fruit, fresh vegetables and fresh seafood, which were in abundance and not of interest to the fearful hoarders. What was indeed sold out in this primarily military town, he said, were all the unhealthy preserved foods like canned and dehydrated goods, because of a perceived military security threat. He derived a general recommendation regarding shopping for food from his experience. "When you visit your local supermarket," he said, "just shop around the outer perimeter where all the good fresh produce is kept. You can omit doing the arduous tour of the inner long aisles. They contain nothing but dead food anyway."

Another physician, Dr. Dong, prescribes reduced meat consumption. His arthritic patients often improve under the dietary restriction. Do you really want to eat all those growth hormones and antibiotics fed to most livestock? The nitrite preservatives in pink meats such as hot dogs, salami and bacon are proven carcinogens.

Advising people to have meat twice a day seems like asking them to ingest a large amount of potentially dangerous chemicals and excess protein. Most eggs are not much better. Those available in supermarkets are mass produced by chickens cooped in dark, cramped cages. The yolks are pale and tasteless. They have probably lost their nutritional value as well. Where in today's huge food stores can you find an egg laid by a hen that has seen daylight even once in her desperate life?

The bread and cereal group is next. We have all seen the bread that most of North America eats. Such a white, false loaf gives little, nutritionally speaking, to the body's cells. The breakfast cereals? Some of them are over 50 percent sugar despite their claims of healthful ingredients only. Don't be fooled by fancy names that only denote more sugar: maltodextrin, glucose, sucrose, lactose, fructose etc. Other clever marketing tries to circumvent consumer-protecting ingredient disclosure laws by describing salt as "sodium."

A parents' group in California has sued Post Cereals for turning children into "sugar junkies." White, unprocessed sugar is in everything from ketchup to crackers. An average Canadian eats over 110 pounds of the "white drug" per year. If he or she is eating the average, "well balanced" diet, it can hardly be avoided. According to Dr. John Yudkin in his book *Sweet and Dangerous*, heart disease, gout and other health problems are now directly linked by several studies to this huge consumption of a chemical not only deficient in itself, but which robs the body of vital nutrients.

Grains like rye, brown rice, and barley are supposed to be part of the bread and cereal group. They are not the standard offering in supermarkets. Bread and flour are usually only white, refined wheat, and if you are lucky, whole wheat. Rice is mainly white. If you ask for any other color, the clerk looks at you as if you are subversive. The supermarkets and food processors have drastically reduced the choice and scope of healthy foods available through their system. Due to them, most consumers are being forced, unwittingly, to forfeit the only pivot on which any diet can balance – variety.

Four servings of the vegetables and fruit group are suggested by the Society. Yet we find produce sprayed with herbicides and pesticides, and grown on mineral-deficient soil. During most of the year, fresh vegetables means brussels sprouts, for example, harvested when still unripe, shipped thousands of miles to be finally cooked into pale submission in a pot of boiling, salted water. The evidence shows that most vitamins do not survive such treatment.

What are we to make of the average diet? It can be extremely harmful, contaminated and a major factor in degenerative diseases such as heart attack, arteriosclerosis, hypertension, stroke, diabetes and cancer. It only seems logical that such a diet be at least investigated as a possible cause of arthritis. Dr. Roger Williams thinks so. "I know of very few people who should be unconcerned about the quality of their food," he writes. "Most physicians seem quite content to accept the Food and Drug Administration's almost meaningless assertion that "vitamins and minerals are supplied in abundant amounts by commonly available foods." [28] Are they indeed?

The Anti-Stress Diet

As we have seen, many researchers believe that some, if not most, types of arthritis are caused by stress – that series of hormone responses preparing you for fight or flight. Think of situations in modern life where it is impossible to react in the way your physical body demands. As a passenger in a fast-moving car, for instance, you might sense danger. Your stress reaction rings the alarm. Your pituitary and adrenal glands generate the hormones priming your body to action. The glands pump and pump, but to no avail, because there you sit quite still and powerless to respond to a situation perceived as threatening by your being.

It is such frustrating inactivity that exhausts the endocrine glands and disturbs your body's internal balance. You may experience similarly frustrating self-denials in work-related exchanges with superiors on whom you perceive yourself to be reliant for survival. In today's urban, densely populated world, physical and mental stressors like these seem unavoidable for the most part. The average so-called "balanced" diet can only aggravate such constant assault on your body's integrity and increases the damage sustained. You need a diet specifically designed to compensate for all that wear and tear. Research has discovered that vitamins C and the B complex are stress protectors of the first order.

Nobel laureate Dr. Linus Pauling claims that vitamin C cures the common cold. Recently, clinical trials conducted by this Nobel laureate and a colleague, Ewan Cameron, at a

Scottish hospital demonstrated that megadoses of the vitamin (10 grams or more per day) significantly prolonged the life span of cancer patients. Dr. Pauling credits such results to the vitamin's ability to increase the body's natural resistance to disease.

Animals under stress can require as much as seventy times the normal requirement of vitamin C to protect the adrenals. Older animals (this analogy has been carried over to older humans) were also found to need twice as much of this vitamin as younger ones. According to Adelle Davis, vitamin C increases the production and utilization of natural cortisone.

Vitamin C is also an important aid to the production of collagen. A marked increase in the permeability of joint tissue cells, due to weak collagen, is often presented in orthodox medical texts as the etiology of several types of arthritis.[29] In 1968, after many studies in this area, Dr. Joseph Chayen of the Kennedy Institute of Rheumatology in Britain reported that enzymes leaking from the cells of the synovial tissue may eat away the cartilage. He recommended large doses of vitamin C to seal up the cell walls. Dr. Pauling has also demonstrated that vitamin C maintains the integrity of connective tissue and is essential for the synthesis of collagen.

Other experiments have shown that a laboratory animal (from a species, which like humans, is unable to manufacture its own vitamin C) on a diet saturated with vitamin C will not reveal any symptoms of arthritis even when injected with bacteria.[30] It is this vitamin which is so vital for the formation of the antibodies that protect against infection.

You can get large amounts of this powerful anti-stressor in organically grown foods such as bean sprouts, rose hips, red and green peppers, cabbage, potatoes, alfalfa and all citrus fruits. If you are arthritic you will probably need especially massive doses, contends Dr. Paavo Airola, both to bolster your natural resistance and, since aspirin is antagonistic to vitamin C, to replace what the painkiller destroys. Many health authorities recommend a natural source supplement of 300 to 500 mg vitamin C taken several times throughout the day. Since this water-soluble vitamin in not stored in the human body, any excess is quickly eliminated. Several smaller doses not only assure a constant supply but reduce the chances of wastage through elimination.

Research has also found the B vitamins extremely effective in overcoming the ravages of stress. "Pantothenic acid (part of the B complex) can scarcely be overemphasized and persons subject to arthritis may have an unusually high requirement for this vitamin. Men deficient in pantothenic acid for only 25 days developed impaired adrenal function," writes Adelle Davis.[31] Carlton Fredericks' studies led him to praise another component of the B complex. "Para-aminobenzoic acid (PABA) makes it possible in some cases to reduce the dose of cortisone in the treatment of arthritis."[32]

Dr. Abram Hoffer, who pioneered orthomolecular psychiatry (the use of large doses of vitamins to overcome mental illness) first used vitamin B3 (niacin) to treat schizophrenia. He discovered it also eradicated many of the symptoms associated with old age, arthritis among them. An article by E.II. Kahan in the *Journal of Orthomolecular Psychiatry* describes this Canadian doctor's successes.

"Dr. Hoffer thought his mother had aged rapidly and was tense and anxious, perhaps due to the serious illness of his father." Before going on an extended business trip, Dr. Hoffer gave his mother pills of niacin and recommended that she take what amounted to three grams daily.

"While in Europe," continues the account, "he received a long letter from her. It was the first time in nearly a year, she wrote, that she was able to hold a pen to write a letter. The swelling in her hands had gone down, the nodules on the joints of her fingers seemed to be disappearing, the pain was much less, and she was able, to her surprise, to hold cups without dropping them and do dishes and other housework without difficulty. She couldn't understand why she was better, but she was overjoyed as, at times, the pain had previously been almost unbearable. This was the first discovery of the use of nicotinic acid (niacin) as a treatment for arthritis. Dr. Hoffer has since prescribed it for other arthritis patients with equally good results." [33]

These three factors, pantothenic acid, PABA and niacin, are just a few of the sixteen known members of the B family. Each of them works in synergy with the others. For this reason an oversupply of one B vitamin can actually cause a deficiency in some of the rest. Therefore, nutritionists advise the use of a vitamin supplement containing the entire B-complex.

Foods most abundant in the B vitamins are brewer's yeast, whole grains, beans and wheat germ. Lecithin, comprised of inositol and choline (part of the B complex) is found in unsaturated vegetable and seed oils as well as in free-range egg yolks. Dr. Carlton Fredericks finds, "Unsaturated fats of the type obtained from wheat germ oil appear also to stimulate pituitary function." [34] Dr. Paavo Airola prefers other types of oils which are more stable such as safflower. He agrees with his colleague about the many health benefits of wheat germ oil, but since it can go rancid very quickly, he advises you use only what you know to be very fresh – not more than a few days old.

Protein is a necessary precursor to the production of ACTH, one of the body's stress hormones. Nutritionists used to recommend liver and other organ meats for stress exhaustion because they are protein-rich. Yet since these foods are related to gout attacks, and may be hormone and drug saturated, it seems sensible to look for other purine-free sources such as organically grown beans and nuts or, if you are not a vegetarian, fresh fish, cheeses made from unpasteurized milk (unfortunately in Canada only foreign, imported cheeses are made from unpasteurized milk!), and free-range eggs available at health food stores. An excellent reference book which shows how to combine meatless protein types to make complete protein meals is *Diet for a Small Planet* by France Moore Lappé.

Protein requirements are not considered to be as high today as they once were. Between 50 to 70 grams a day is considered sufficient for arthritics by the respected German physician, Ernst Schneider, MD, while Dr. Airola advises even less and emphasizes vegetable sources.

Stress draws calcium from the bones. High amounts of the mineral then freely circulate in the bloodstream to eventually be deposited at weak spots like the soft tissues surrounding a joint. The result is the formation of nodules and bony spurs at bone ends. Extra supplementation is necessary with calcium and/or silica (indispensable for all connective tissue growth cycles) and vitamin D (which together with silica aids in calcium metabolism) and vitamin E (which in combination with silica prevents the calcification of soft tissues).

The researchers just quoted maintain that if calcium is constantly extracted from your bones without being replaced, you will end up with osteoporosis (loss of bone density) and consequently the weak, easily breakable bones so common in old age. Latest research indicates that increased silica intake may be the answer to preventing osteoporosis, calcium loss, and a host of other ailments affecting the connective tissues so sensitive in arthritis patients. However, silica's general healing and restorative powers are too vast and broad to be addressed here.[35]

When stress is caused by tension, emotional upheaval, and suppressed resentment, the doyenne of nutrition writers

Cathryn Elwood suggests the nerve-calming minerals calcium and magnesium plus soy bean lecithin and the essential fatty acids of cold pressed vegetable and seed oils.

Here's a quick review of some foods that can help or hinder.

Enemies (to be avoided constantly):
- white sugar
- white processed flour and bread
- cakes and pastries
- tea and coffee
- processed foods of all descriptions
- alcohol

Friends (use these every day):
- raw foods and fruit juices
- whole grains
- cold-pressed vegetable and seed oils
- all the vitamins, but particularly C and B complex
- calcium and magnesium
- silica
- alfalfa sprouts
- parsley
- garlic
- comfrey
- sour cherries
- pineapples
- brewer's yeast
- cod liver oil

The Anti-Allergy Diet

As you may have suspected, such a diet has to be individualized. An anti-allergy diet must take into account highly personal food sensitivities. There is therefore no generalized approach possible. A good beginning is an allergy test. This is best preceded by a fast (see Fasting for Relief) and a carefully monitored elimination diet. This means that certain foods, suspected of causing the allergy that in turn causes the food-induced arthritis, should be left out of the diet. In his book *Lifetime Arthritis Relief System*, Marshall Mandell, MD, prescribes a Six-Day Rotary Diagnostic Diet, which, unlike an elimination diet, intentionally introduces foods for diagnostic purposes to which you may be sensitive.

Experimental case studies have proven that food-induced arthritis is a fact of life for some people. Sufferers should undergo allergy testing. You may follow Dr. Mandell's diagnostic diet but I would suggest that, in most cases, food allergy diets are best conducted under the professional guidance of a nutritional physician or counselor. This reduces the possible margin for error.

Allergy, broadly speaking, is a lack of body resistance to certain irritants, and there are very many possible irritants. For this reason, the cause of allergy-induced arthritis lies in the individual and not in the environment and also not in the nutrients as such. Arthritis-related allergy studies undertaken in the late eighties in Switzerland and India confirmed that, while certain foods do make the symptoms worse, there is no food item common to food allergies. Before embarking on extensive and expensive testing however, you may want to first try out the other recommendations of this chapter. By following them rigorously, you may find that your allergy problem has been taken care of.

Healing by Nutrients

While vitamins and minerals are found as nutrients in our food, because of their importance, they are discussed under their own heading. (See Vitamins and Minerals below.)

Food analysis is getting better at not only identifying individual nutrients in foods, but also classifying them according to their effects, and if they are useful, synthesizing them for therapy. One such nutrient is phenylalanine, an amino acid. It is the precursor of the amino acid tyrosine that cannot be reconverted by the body. Because of this inability, phenylalanine is essential to the diet.

The DL- form of phenylalanine has been successfully used in clinical practice as a natural pain reliever in all forms of arthritis. DL-phenylalanine does not work all the time, is not a complete therapy, and does not treat the underlying causes. It is, however, a psychoactive remedy that can also uplift mood. DL-phenylalanine can be taken in doses of 500 to 750 mg two to three times daily.

DL-phenylalanine should not be taken for longer than three weeks at a time. If you are interested in it as a temporary dietary, supplement for pain relief, you should know that for best performance, phenylalanine metabolism requires the vitamins pyridoxine (B6), niacin (B3), and C and the minerals copper and iron. It is probably also a good idea to take it together with all the other synergistically working amino acids. If taken alone, even though generally free of side effects, it should be taken while under the care of a qualified nutritionist, naturopath or other expert in nutritional medicine because its catecholamine effect could raise blood pressure in susceptible individuals.[36] Depending on where you live, you may also not be able to purchase it in isolated form because of restrictions. This is currently true in Canada, but is being fought by the health food industry.

The sulfur-containing, non-essential amino acid cysteine is found in foods like poultry, yogurt, oats, wheat germ, egg yolks, red peppers, garlic, onions, broccoli and brussels sprouts. In the L-form, that is, L-cysteine, it is indicated by Elson M. Haas, MD as a natural nutritional treatment for fighting inflammation in rheumatoid arthritis.[37] Ranges of 250 to 750 mg daily taken in several portions throughout the day are indicated. L-cysteine should be taken with three times as much vitamin C to prevent crystallization of excess cystine, another amino acid to which L-cysteine can be converted in the body.

Another important supplement in arthritis management is evening primrose oil. The seed of the evening primrose yields an oil that contains gamma-linolenic acid (GLA). This oil is a precursor of the important prostaglandin E1 series (PGE1). Most GLA research stems from England. The findings indicate that evening primrose oil is of great benefit in clearing or reducing the symptoms of arthritis and other inflammatory conditions.

Our bodies can make gamma-linolenic acid from linoleic acid and then convert it to the prostaglandin E1 series. This series is probably the most important of the hormone-like prostaglandins. Among a wide range of metabolic benefits, these substances help inhibit or reduce inflammation in rheumatoid arthritis while boosting the immune system and correcting possible GLA and EFA deficiencies that may contribute to the occurrence of arthritic inflammations. Although the use of evening primrose oil is still experimental, the future looks promising. Dr. Haas claims especially good pain-reduction for arthritic patients when evening primrose oil therapy is boosted by vitamin E and beta-carotene (vitamin A) with side effects basically nonexistent especially when taken with food.[38]

On the assumption that oil, in general, would make a natural joint lubricant, a team of doctors treated arthritic patients with cod liver oil. Dr. Charles A. Brusch reported on the therapy in the *Journal of the National Medical Association* (July 1959). Each day the patients drank a glass of water one hour before breakfast or half an hour before dinner. Milk or warm soup was the only liquid allowed with meals. Cod liver oil, mixed thoroughly with either a small amount of orange juice or milk, was taken on an empty stomach either four hours after the last meal of the day or one hour before breakfast. The physicians also insisted on a "complete curtailment of soft drinks, candy, cake, ice cream or any goods made up of white sugar."

Within several months the overwhelming majority (ninety-two out of ninety-eight patients) responded with marked reduction in pain and a general improvement in mobility. This program, although essentially designed for osteo-arthritics, might also be helpful to rheumatoid sufferers, Dr. Brusch emphasized, because of its ability to correct faulty body chemistry and promote good health. For instance, elevated cholesterol and blood pressure levels dropped for all those on the cod liver oil treatment. For a further and more detailed explanation of the exact way to carry out this therapy in your own home, I suggest the book *Arthritis and Common Sense* by Dale Alexander.

Cod liver oil, however, should not be overused, cautions Dr. Haas, because it is too high in vitamins A and D, and because the livers of fish concentrate toxic materials the fish may have absorbed. He points instead to the therapeutic use of eicosapentaenoic acid and decosahexaenoic acid (EPA and DHA), exciting fatty acid nutrients found in fish that have become very popular recently. EPA and DHA exhibit a mild anti-inflammatory effect and are therefore useful in arthritis treatment. The treatment with EPA and DHA, according to Dr. Haas, is enhanced by eating cold water fish like salmon, trout, herring, mackerel or sardines, or by taking additional oil supplements.

Among seafoods, New Zealand green-lipped mussel extracts have been found to be particularly effective in alleviating arthritis. This treatment was used by the world-famous heart surgeon Dr. Christian Barnard, a sufferer from arthritis. He talks about it in his *Program for Living with Arthritis*.

An Alkaline Diet of Raw Foods and Juices

Everyone knows that fresh fruit and vegetables are essential to a healthy diet. But when your body is sick and infected, as happens in arthritis, a cleansing and restorative regime of raw foods and juices is doubly necessary.

The value behind such a diet is its ability to reduce the acidity of the bloodstream, and increase its alkalinity. The result is a more soothing pH. Most processed foods, meats, starches and sugars – even grains, seeds and dried beans – are acid-forming, while vegetables and fruits are alkaline. Citrus fruits which contain acid are metabolized in such a way that they take on a neutral pH. Apple cider vinegar, a popular folk remedy for rheumatic aches, is similarly transformed.

According to Paavo Airola's teachings, a raw foods or vegetable diet emphasizing alfalfa, wheat grass, watercress, potatoes (cooked and raw), celery, parsley, garlic, comfrey and endive is recommended. Such a regime is full of fiber and helps to prevent constipation. If food residues are retained in the colon for longer than the regular and safe twenty-four hour transit time, they become a source of acidity. Overeating is discouraged, and with the sweets and starches reduced, one naturally tends to lose weight on this diet. Unnecessary pounds further burden weakened joints, and many doctors will advise arthritics to reduce. Thus on the alkaline diet, you can safely, and even deliciously, solve several disease-inducing problems at once.

Dr. Howard Hay, a well known authority on arthritis, attributes the ailment to salts caused by an acid-forming diet. "Urates" [39] he claims, "are actually outside the circulation, deposited in the free joint cavity, and are not usually absorbable, and thus constitute a permanent crippling." [40]

Hay agrees with the Airola teaching that the diet must be changed to an alkaline-forming one. But, he warns those accustomed to "quick-fix drugs," the results are not immediate, or even, in the short run, pleasant. "It is not unusual to have a marked aggravation of the arthritis after you first begin changing the body's chemistry, and this is caused not by anything you are eating, but by chemicals already stored in your body that are still being precipitated. Go on with your new diet for a number of weeks and you will find the condition arrested, for the pain is less and the attacks of acute arthritis less frequent and less severe."[41]

Additions to a raw foods diet, which some claim have brought them relief, are goat's milk and sour cherries. Brome-lain, an enzyme obtained from pineapple has proven effective in reducing swelling and inflammation. For a thorough cleansing and elimination of the built-up toxins, Airola recommends a juice fast. "All rheumatic diseases," he said, "including rheumatoid arthritis, are particularly responsive to vegetable juice therapy. The alkaline action of raw juices and vegetable broth dissolves the accumulation of deposits around the joints and in other tissues."

The length of a fast depends on your general state of health and the severity of the disease. Many people prefer to fast under the supervision of a naturopath or physician who sympa-thizes with this age-old (in Europe at least) treatment. For complete instructions on juice fasting and a matchless personal guide for beginners read *The Joy of Juice Fasting – for Health, Cleansing & Weight Loss* by Klaus Kaufmann. You can find the book in health food stores and selected book stores.

Former arthritics say they successfully combined fasting with the raw foods program. A young-looking grandmother claimed she had excellent results when she went on a short (eight-day) juice fast. This, she said, accelerated the elimination of toxins from her body. She then concentrated on a raw foods diet, no bread or cooked food of any description. She also took large doses of the anti-stress vitamins and added wheat germ to her salads, and brewer's yeast to her morning juice.

The stiffness and pain she had felt, off and on, for over a year, in her fingers and shoulder completely disappeared after a month and a half. She could not believe that some kind of throbbing wouldn't start up again, especially as the cold and rainy fall weather had started, yet there was no recurrence. That it had taken so many weeks of what she called 'rabbit food' disheartened her. She looked forward to something warm. The ailment may have taken fifty years to create, so obviously couldn't vanish overnight.

After a few more weeks on raw foods, she began to slowly add other foods back into her menu – whole grains, nuts, seeds, unprocessed cheeses from unpasteurized milk and similar dairy products. To this day she has completely refrained from what used to be such a large part of each meal for her – refined starches, desserts, white sugar and processed foods. She says she now knows the true healing path, and never again will she venture from it.

Detoxification Diet

A detoxification diet is a most subtle medicine that instills positive changes on many levels. Leaving out the white sugar and processed foods is certainly a great beginning for any detoxification. Eating only fresh, certified organically-grown foods is the best way to avoid toxin build up and start a detoxification diet. Watch food labels and do not purchase foods that contain the following additives: artificial color, sodium nitrite, sodium nitrate, BHT (butylated hydroxy-toluene), saccharin, sulphite (sodium bisulfate), sulfur dioxide, BVO (brominated vegetable oil).

Perhaps the detoxification process should begin even before we are getting toxins into our actual food items. Take a look at your cooking utensils and, if possible, eliminate those made of aluminum. Although there is no hard evidence about the aluminum hazards, in case of arthritics, it is probably the best policy not to take chances. A good alternative is cooking ware made of stainless steel.

There are a number of other toxic and heavy metals that we must be sure to eliminate as far as possible to avoid overexposure. Aluminum, for instance, also occurs in certain food additives like processed cheese, white flour and common table salt. Antacids, which many people take, often contain aluminum hydroxide.

Avoiding weed killers and insecticides in your home will make sure that you avoid overexposure to arsenic. Avoiding eating shell fish and drinking tap water may help in reducing cadmium intake, as will not smoking and avoiding coffee and black tea, which may contain significant amounts of cadmium. It is interesting that there is absolutely no cadmium in newborn babies. Cadmium is prevented from crossing into the placenta. However, cadmium accumulates in tissues (other than brain tissue) with age.

Unfortunately, lead exposure and levels of lead in the body are higher in North America than anywhere else in the world. Non-organically grown grains and legumes and commercial, non-organic fruit and vegetables contain some lead. Processed meats, especially sausages, are even higher in lead. Tap water often contains significant amounts of lead (and/or copper, an excess of which is connected to schizophrenia).

Eating canned foods can result in lead intake as the solder holding the seams together is very often made of lead. Other sources are cosmetics, tobacco products (one more thing against smoking!) and pesticides. Lead-containing glazes on pottery are another problem and food should not be stored, cooked or served in such containers. Jogging along much-traveled roadsides is another lead hazard. Joggers who run along traffic-congested roads, exercise their lungs and fill them with exhaust fumes – sheer insanity! Luckily, all of these hazards can be easily avoided.

You may have mercury in your teeth if you have so-called silver amalgam fillings. The 1991 booklet *Eliminating Poison in Your Mouth* provides more on this subject. Its up-to-date findings will surprise you. Despite the American Food and Drug Administration's recent avowal that mercury fillings are not dangerous, there is no doubt that mercury is a virulent poison much like nicotine and should be avoided whenever possible. Other metals to avoid are barium (used in x-ray evaluations) and beryllium (in industrial and rocket fuel).

Finally, anything that intensifies our processes of elimination (breathing, sweating, urinating, defecating), constitutes a detoxification. Exercising to a sweat will get rid of poisons under the skin. Drinking plenty of fresh spring water will certainly help to detoxify our body. Eating plenty of roughage to induce regular bowel movements will detoxify the digestive tract.

Fasting for Relief

This is a good way of beginning the body's detoxification process and it happens to help arthritis. Even though scientific double-blind studies of dietary effects on arthritis sufferers have not been totally satisfactory (often because of unwilling subjects and puzzling placebo effects), fasting periods show that arthritis almost always improves in the absence of food. During 1988, Swedish rheumatologists found that fasting reduces the disease activity in rheumatoid arthritis. They therefore suggested that brief periods of fasting may be used to bring about rapid improvement during flare-ups.[42]

It seems that fasting changes the blood chemistry of people with arthritis.[43] Fasting slows the action of certain enzymes and blocks key steps in the sequence that leads to inflammation. Studies have shown that people do not suffer untoward side effects from controlled fasting, especially juice fasting, other than weight loss, passing weakness and lightheadedness. If you are interested in undertaking a self-guided fasting program, I would recommend following the juice fasting rules in *The Joy of Juice Fasting*.

Unlike most fasting methods, you will not be deprived of essential nutrients during such a juice fast. The book provides excellent recipes for preparing for a fast as well as providing for balanced after-fast meals to ease return to a regular diet.

Vitamins and Minerals

As pointed out previously, vitamin A has been successfully used in treating arthritis. Vitamin E, often recommended for connective tissue repair, has been found to be anti-inflammatory in conditions like bursitis, gout and arthritis. Another fat-soluble vitamin may help arthritic patients because of its ability to reduce irritation in the synovial linings of the joints. This is vitamin K, found in nature mostly in alfalfa, but also in other foods.

Vitamin K derived from food sources is known as phylloquinone or K1. Our intestinal bacteria produce another K vitamin, K2 or menaquinone. A synthetic form of this vitamin, K3 is twice as active as the two natural forms and may be of particular help for people with decreased bile secretion who do not metabolize the two natural vitamin Ks very well.

We have previously discussed Dr. Hoffer's use of niacin on his mother. Niacin or vitamin B3 has been found to sometimes be of benefit in arthritis treatment, probably because of its ability to stimulate blood flow to the capillaries. Nicotinic acid, the "flushing" form of niacin, should be employed in arthritis treatment rather than the niacinamide form which does not produce the well-known skin flush that results from the capillary action. [44]

Another important B vitamin, pantothenic acid or vitamin B5 is the anti-stress (adrenal support) vitamin. I have detailed its beneficial use in arthritis under the Anti-Stress Diet heading above. B12 or cobalamin, however, deserves mention as it has been found useful in the treatment of osteoarthritis.[45] Ascorbic acid or vitamin C has been discussed thoroughly throughout this book and under the heading of Anti-Stress Diet above because its effects are so all-pervasive. Its beneficial influence on cortisone and collagen deserves repeating because both are so intimately connected to arthritis.

Minerals are important and most often work synergistically with the vitamins. The highly respected discoverer of pantothenic acid, Dr. Roger Williams, explains why minerals are of such importance to health, but especially for preventing osteoarthritis. "Many of the difficulties associated with arthritis diseases," he writes, "stem from what in popular terms we may call poor lubrication. Our joints and all other movable structures in our bodies must be lubricated, and the lubricant commonly used is called 'synovial fluid.' This is a viscous (sticky), mostly dilute water solution of various minerals, but contains one percent of mucinous protein (muco-protein) that gives it lubricating properties... The lubricating quality of synovial fluid is certain to be greatly influenced by the minerals that are in it, and it is quite conceivable that in some individuals the arthritic condition may be largely due to inappropriate mineral balance."[46]

Minerals are also needed to neutralize poisonous acid-forming waste collected in the body. By combining with the toxins they thus prepare them for elimination. "Were it not for minerals, waste products would accumulate in the body and create toxic reactions that could be fatal," reports the nutritionist Carlson Wade.[47] The two most essential minerals linked with arthritis prevention by the two authorities just quoted are calcium and magnesium. Both are found in green leafy vegetables and are available in tablet form.

According to Dr. Howland, it is also important to make sure that there is enough zinc in the diet. This can be achieved simply by taking three 10 mg zinc tablets per day in the form of either zinc sulfate or zinc gluconate.[48]

Healthy Cooking

It is clear by now that healthy food is the key to well-being. I have described all of the nutrients that will help fight off arthritis. Now, with a little bit of imagination and a penchant for cooking we can not only keep arthritis at bay, but have a tasty meal too. The recipes following (always for one person) are only meant to stimulate your own kitchen talents in accordance with the nutrient requirements outlined in this book:

Potatoes and Onions

    2 potatoes
    5 onions
    1 tablespoon parsley
    1 tablespoon Vegit

Wash and slice potatoes and onions. Add parsley and seasoning and cook for 15 minutes in 1 cup of water. It is simply delicious.

Salmon Delight

    1 piece of fresh salmon, preferably a centre cut
    1 large onion
    2 carrots
    fresh parsley
    seasoning

Wash and dry the salmon, rub with seasoning, place in closed baking dish or foil, add vegetables by arranging around the salmon. Bake in the oven at 350 degrees for about 10 minutes. Garnish with fresh parsley, sliced almonds and lemon wedges and serve. Delightful!

My Caesar Salad

       1/2 fresh, organically grown romaine lettuce, washed, torn by hand into bite-sized pieces

       1 fresh anchovy fillet, sliced

       1 crushed garlic clove

       1/4 tsp mustard

       1 slice flax seed bread toasted and cut into cubes

       juice of 1/4 lemon

       1 tsp grated parmesan cheese

       1 tsp fresh cold-pressed flax oil

       1 free range egg yolk

Place anchovy pieces, garlic and mustard into a mortar. Add a few toasted bread cubes to assist crushing. Using the pestle, crush and mash ingredients into a thick, smooth paste. If the ingredients are well smoothed, the dressing will be light and creamy. Now add lemon juice and egg yolk and carefully fold under. Add parmesan, then oil and beat smooth. Toss salad before serving and add the remaining croutons. Magnifico!

Meatless Meat sauce

Get, from your health food store or organic green grocer, a selection of many fresh vegetables, always one each, for example:

       1 carrot,

       1 green pepper

       1 red pepper

       1 yellow pepper

1 asparagus
1 segment of broccoli
1 of cauliflower
1 small turnip
1 potato
1 onion
1 garlic
1 shallot
1 kohlrabi
1 celery stick
1 sweet potato
1 tomato
1 radish
1 string bean
1 tsp each dried, organically-grown legumes: peas,
    beans, lentils
1 tsp each dried unsalted organically-grown nuts:
    almonds, cashews, filberts, brazil nuts
1 tsp unsalted, cultured European butter
tomato paste
seasonings

Cut and slice all vegetables into bite-sized pieces. Melt butter in a large skillet and sauté onions for a few minutes. Reduce heat, add all vegetables and steam for a few minutes. Add cold fresh spring water and all legumes. Cover and let simmer for 60 minutes. Stir in tomato paste and add seasonings to taste. I usually put in the whole larder, but leave out the salt. Add your favorite pasta and enjoy!

Spring Soup

Use the same ingredients as for meatless meat sauce above; excepting the tomato paste.

Prepare and cook as before, but leave out the tomato paste

and add more water. You can easily find other suitable vegetables, dried vegetables (legumes), nuts, etc. to add to this kaleidoscope of spring. This makes a great-tasting, excellent meal by itself and puts lots of clean green energy into your body.

6

Other Pain-Relieving Methods

Rest and Exercise

When your arthritis flares up, the only thing you probably want to do is lie in bed. Many doctors say that is the best immediate treatment for acute attacks. Not only the rest for your body, but that afforded to your mind, is particularly healing. Even between those painful bouts, it is recommended that you remain flat on your back, knees and head straight, arms at your sides, for at least an hour longer than you might normally each night. If possible, put your feet up for a while each afternoon as well.

Yet, as with most things, rest can be overdone. Even though joints are aching they need to be used or further stiffness may ensue. The muscles too must be kept limber through some form of mild exercise. The balance between activity and repose is difficult to achieve for anyone, and for the arthritis sufferer it has to be worked out on an individual basis through trial and error.

How severe is the pain? How good is mobility? What is your age? What is your medical history? How is your cholesterol level? How is your heart? All these and so many other factors have to be weighed against the potential benefits of physical exertion. Ask your own (ideally wholistically-minded) doctor to help develop a program designed for your strengths and needs. Meanwhile, the following are simple, relaxing exercises you can do throughout the day. By all means, however, don't push yourself. Build up your repertoire of bends and stretches gradually.

Walking: Brisk walking out-of-doors is a good warm-up for all the muscles. It also stimulates the respiratory and circulatory systems. You'll find your body relaxing and tension evaporating as you walk. At last you are doing what all those stress hormones are secreted for: responding physically.

While out on these little jaunts psychologists advise noticing the things around you. Feel the sunshine or the gray clouds, listen to the birds, the traffic or the muffled sounds in snow. It may even happen, and it usually does, that those interior pain signals grow less strident as you become more aware of what is going on around you. At any rate, you are bound to feel a little more cheerful by getting out of the house. If you think you need an impetus, no doubt your own or the neighbor's dog would love to be taken for a stroll.

Stretching: Stand straight, feet together. Stretch slowly and gently until your fingers touch the floor. Bend your knees if you want (we are not training for the Olympics) and then straighten slowly, trying to touch the ceiling. Repeat this as often as feels comfortable. This relaxing activity will loosen and stretch many muscles through your back and legs.

Head Swirl: Let your head go limp on your neck. Slowly rotate it in a complete circle from right to left several times, then reverse direction and repeat. Let your shoulders also go limp. Slowly, easily are the key words here.

Arm Swing: Bend at the waist so that your upper body is at a right angle to your legs. Let your arms dangle. Relax the neck and back muscles. Now swing each arm back and forth in a soothing rhythm.

Arm Circles: Hold both arms out to the sides at shoulder height with palms up. Trace small backward circles ten times. Repeat with palms down and reverse the circular motion.

Swimming: Special mention must be made of swimming as potentially the most restorative exercise. This is true at least of swimming in clean safe rivers, lakes, and the ocean or supervised pools fed by such natural bodies of water. Unfortunately, many of today's public pools contain high concentrations of chlorine that may nullify any health benefit of exercise by exposure to poisonous chlorine. I advise you to check out the chlorine levels at your local pool by calling the pool administration before taking the plunge.

After you can complete the above exercises, there are many other easy-to-do exercises you can fit into your daily exercise program.

Massage Therapy

Massage therapy is based on touching and manipulating muscles. Touching is one of the most pain-alleviating things. A friendly touch on the shoulder reassures a friend and alleviates the pain of a child. It has been proven by scientific research that sexual activity, an intimate form of touching, greatly helps to reduce arthritic pains. It is hardly surprising then, that both self-massage and professional massage therapy will help to reduce arthritic pain.

Hand-held electric massagers are soothing as are vibrator pillows, chairs, and beds. Not everyone can afford these luxuries, but most people suffering from arthritis can obtain medicare-covered sessions with a registered massage therapist, which is probably the better way to go about getting a massage in any event. After all, the therapist knows exactly how to find the right spots for applying pressure and the right muscles to massage and relax around the inflamed joints.

If you do not know a registered massage therapist (do not confuse massage therapy with physiotherapy!), get a referral from your family doctor. You may need one anyway to qualify for medicare reimbursement. With some orthodox-minded doctors, you may have to insist a little harder before they relent and issue a referral. If your doctor refuses altogether to prescribe massage therapy, it may be time for you to find a new family physician who is more modern in his or her thinking.

Alternatively, self-massage may be employed. A light lubricant cream or oil should be applied to the area to be massaged. Use light strokes in the direction of the heart while applying suitable pressure with your finger tips, thumbs and the heel of the hand. You may also employ loofahs and massage brushes in order to stimulate skin circulation.

Heliotherapy

Warm weather and sunshine, in fact heat from most sources, has a palliative effect on arthritic pain. Particularly soothing can be deep-penetrating infrared lamps. Natural sunlight, has a particular physiological benefit provided it is controlled and sunburn is avoided. Artificial sun lamps, however, should be shunned. Up to half an hour in the sun is considered healthful provided exposure is gradually increased from just a few minutes.

Ultraviolet rays combine with the oils on the skin's surface to form ergosterol. This is then absorbed through the epidermis and converted into vitamin D, the pivotal component in proper calcium absorption by the bloodstream and in turn, the bones. Artificial white light slightly aids vitamin D synthesis, but beware of ordinary fluorescent light. It can deplete your much-needed stores of the vitamin. Fluorescent bulbs, if any, should be full spectrum lights. These healthful lights are available through your health food store or (in Canada) from Flora Distributors in Burnaby, BC.

John Ott, PhD, a researcher into the effects of light, describes what happened to his arthritis after six months of conscious exposure to natural sunshine. "Suddenly, I didn't seem to need the cane... My hip hadn't felt this well for three or four years. I began walking back and forth awhile. I ran into the house, up stairs two at a time, to tell my wife." [49]

Hydrotherapy

Water is one of the most soothing of all mediums. Whether you are in a bathtub at home or in a therapeutic pool, the water supports, floats and soothes your afflicted joints. Once the pressure of gravity is thus greatly reduced, you can naturally move with much less effort and pain. Water immersion, no matter if you are just relaxing or actively swimming or exercising, is called hydrotherapy. It stimulates circulation which means, in turn, an increased elimination of the toxins which normally tend to accumulate in a sluggish blood-stream.

Applied heat expands the blood vessels. Thus hot water therapy is particularly effective in encouraging trapped poisons to pass through and out of the system. The simple luxury of a warm bath every day will ease stiff joints immeasurably. It can be very enervating. However, hydrotherapists caution against staying in any longer than thirty minutes at high temperature. After the bath a brisk toweling will further accelerate blood flow.

Most of the famous spas of Europe attach great regenerative powers to alternating hot and cold baths. This water cure, first originated by the German champion of water therapy, Father Kneipp, will stimulate the body functions, especially the adrenal and endocrine glands, and reactivate their functions.

You do not have to travel to an alpine spa to get this invigorating treatment. At home, take a hot shower for three to five minutes. This will warm up the body. Then rapidly switch to cold water for a few seconds. The contrast will almost take your breath away. Let the cold water fall first on the right side of your body, away from your heart. Repeat this for three turns, ending with cold water. Finish with an energetic toweling. Dry-brushing your entire body with a loofah is also recommended by Father Kneipp, to promote circulation.

Cryotherapy

This is also known as cold treatment and involves the application of ice. Cryotherapy is best employed in conjunction with heat therapy (see Hydrotherapy and Heliotherapy above and Hot Wax Therapy below). The idea here is that what the heat won't alleviate, the ice will anaesthetize. Alternating hot and cold (iced) water baths are one excellent way of employing cryotherapy.

Obviously the general health of the arthritic patient must be considered before using cryotherapy. In most cases, however, ice or cold sprays will soothe inflamed joints. Care should be taken to avoid frosting the skin or causing deep cold ache. Briefly chilling the tissues over and around a joint, and then stretching the tissues by slow movement can achieve improved movement and pain reduction.

Hot Wax Therapy

This home treatment is lengthy and cumbersome, but it really works to relieve pain, particularly in the hands and wrists. Melt paraffin wax, mixed with a few drops of mineral water, in the top of a double boiler. Wax is very flammable and should not be heated over a direct source. Remove from the stove and allow to cool until a thick white coating forms on the top. One at a time, dip your hands, up to the wrists, quickly into the wax and just as rapidly, out again. Repeat this a few more times, allowing the wax to cool on your skin between applications.

To retain the soothing heat, you can wrap your coated hand in toweling or a plastic bag. For larger joints, melted wax can be applied with a paint brush. After it has lost its heat, the wax may easily be peeled off and re-used indefinitely.

Magnetic Mending

Here is an opportunity to get away from aspirin and other drugs for pain control. Electromagnetic healing is a totally safe form of pain relief through cellular stimulation. The method employs a small electromagnetic field that is generated by a battery-driven unit.[50] The concept of magnetic field therapy is not all that new, however, older electromagnetic devices were often too large or too expensive for individual self-help.

Electromagnetic stimulation can be very effective in pain control according to studies performed in Germany and Austria. A 1968 study done in Munich by Dr. Lechner documents the results of 642 cases of induced arthrosis in which substantial improvements had taken place through the implementation of magnetic field therapy.

An electrobiological stimulant generates a pulsating, low-frequency magnetic field in the 2-24 Hz range. For arthritic pain control, the device is generally set to operate at 10-15 Hz during the day and 2-10 Hz during the night. However, individual settings can be varied in a range from 2-24 Hz. Applied to the affected parts of the body, the low-frequency field generates currents in the living cells of the affected area.

This causes subtle changes in the cell membrane and alleviates pain.

The beauty of this pain relieving method is that it can be employed any time and together with any other therapy, as magnetic healing is supplementary therapy. Magnetic field therapy is, however, not suitable for people with heart pacemakers, during pregnancy or problems with psychic disorders, or immediately following myocardial infarction (heart attack). For anyone else however, electromagnetic field therapy offers a chance to escape the potential adverse side effects of anti-inflammatory drugs.

7

Rejuvenation
Can Conquer Arthritis

Longevity Diet

There's no such thing, right? Wrong – by following the dietary advice for longevity, you can do more than free yourself from the pain of arthritis, you can actually add precious years to your newly precious life. Adult aging, aside from the mere count of the years, involves the degeneration of body systems. A diet and lifestyle selected for anti-aging factors automatically promises arthritic relief as well, because, as pointed out in the introduction, arthritis is often a degenerative disease, and, degeneration and aging do not necessarily have to go together.

We are looking for something that will enhance our immune system, allow us to tolerate greater stress, prevent cancer and arteriosclerosis (the disease behind cardiovascular disease), maintain sexual vitality and keep our skin in shape. What can best help to achieve all of this? While it is basically very simple, the simple is often the most difficult to implement. Consider the example of smokers who know smoking is unhealthy but often enough find themselves unable to do the simple thing of quitting.

If you don't make the necessary dietary changes, be prepared to live a "normal," statistically average life span of (in 1993) 70 to 80 years. Modern medical and scientific advances are usually able to keep patients living, even if they are full of pain and misery. By following the longevity diet, however, you should be able to be alive at age 100 and feel good about it. So, with a toast to the future, happy centenarians, here is the longevity diet. It is up to you to implement it.

1. Eat less – always under-eat. Stop eating while you still feel hungry. Avoid obesity. Eat low-calorie foods, such as fresh fruit or vegetables.
2. Eat dietary fiber – roughage helps elimination.
3. Reduce fat intake – even consumption of cold-pressed vegetable oils should be minimized.
4. Eat complex carbohydrates – lots of whole grains, legumes, potatoes, squash.
5. Moderate protein intake – select nuts, seeds, whole grains and legumes as your proteins over meats, fish, eggs and dairy products.
6. Do not eat chemical additives – this basically means no cured or prepared meats, but check labels and do not even purchase items that contain chemicals.
7. Avoid salt, sugar, alcohol, nicotine, and caffeine. The worst offender is nicotine. Remember that even honey is sugar.
8. Drink lots of pure spring water. Avoid any water that has additives (most tap water).
9. Detoxify your system from time to time by going on a cleansing or juice fast. Twice a year (spring and fall) is a good idea.
10. Supplement – ignore the health authorities that tell

you otherwise. Don't listen to their well-meant advice, even if it is supported by your regular doctor. Fortify your diet with vitamins and minerals. All antioxidants help to maintain cellular tissues. You can get the recommended dosages from your nutrition-oriented medical doctor, naturopath or nutritionist, who can tailor a supplement program to your needs.

The following dietary supplements may be part of such a program: Vitamin E, beta-carotene (better than vitamin A), vitamin C, selenium (best is selenomethionine), L-cysteine, zinc, manganese, copper, silica (organic or gel), calcium, magnesium, chromium, molybdenum, niacin, vitamin B12, folic acid, RNA, choline, flaxseed oil, L-carnitine, coenzyme Q10 (ubiquinone), lactobacillus acidophilus, organic germanium, mucopolysaccharides (chondroitin sulphates), digestive enzymes (where required), garlic, ginseng, cayenne (capsicum), gotu kola, wheat germ oil, vitamin K, B-complex, bioflavonoids, L-amino acids complex.

Happiness Is ...

Diet, exercise, water and heat all have their place in a total program to overcome arthritis. But what can often help most is a tranquil and happy state of mind. Impossible, you think? The terrible, physical reality of pain can easily lead to such depression, resentment and feelings of being trapped that the mere idea of contentment seems like a dream.

But many experts believe that your ailment is very likely stress-induced. Many studies have found that the stressors are frustration, constant tension and repressed hostility. Adapt your philosophy to the circumstances of your life, stress researchers suggest. That doesn't mean you need not strive or try to change your situation. "Only don't," as Dr. Selye advises, "put up resistance in vain." You'll just be increasing your tension.

The total or wholistic approach lives up to its name. Orthomolecular psychiatry has proven that the proper nutritional environment for brain cells can overcome depression. Exercise promotes relaxation. Both proper nutrition and exercise work to encourage a happier, less tense disposition. Such an attitude then completes the circle – it's both the prerequisite and the result of feeling better.

J.I. Rodale, one of the original promoters of preventive health care in the US, agreed that good spirits help good health. In the magazine he started, *Prevention*, he wrote, "There is a place for seriousness. But a good laugh is a means of staying healthy. It will empty stale air out of one's lungs. In other words, just as one should get so many milligrams of vitamin C every day, so should one attempt to do a certain amount of laughing every day."

It's a good idea. It certainly can't do any of us harm. We may even discover a certain release and self forgetfulness in good humor and brave thoughts.

Believing in Immortality – A Positive Outlook

It is hard to imagine permanence in a world where change is the obvious motor force and death is commonplace. Despite major religions and the many minor cults that offer their individual views of eternity, there is a cold hell out there for many people who simply cannot see the forest for the trees.

Religion, however, is not the subject of this book – healing arthritis is! But, a spiritual belief in immortality is an absolute prerequisite for a healthy human being. Whether that belief in immortality is of the body (through children, or exemption from death), of the mind (undying fame of the kind Plato, Shakespeare, Michelangelo and Mozart achieved), or of the spirit (the soul, the eternal essence of man, ascending) or of all three, the important thing for maintaining a healthy attitude is to foster a belief in the eternal.

We must believe that our soul-life is eternal. There comes a point in life when, in regarding the world around us, we realize that none of it is of any value unless there is immortality. Reason is only a partial discovery of what is, and will fail us in our search for immortality. It failed even the greatest thinkers! Belief on faith takes over where reason ends. So, whether you are ready or not, you must believe. Believe in God. Believe in your own eternalness and, if you must have a reason: because it feels better. So develop your belief system with daily prayer or meditation, make sure it is belief in goodness and in what feels good, and you are half-way there. Belief that you will heal your arthritis is rejuvenation of the spirit – the body will follow the spirit!

The Story Doesn't End Here

The conventional approach claims that aspirin and other dangerous drugs are the best medicines. This is, at best, narrow and one-sided. The family practitioners really can't be blamed. Most often they are confronted with a crisis. A patient comes to them in agony and desperation, demanding immediate relief – something "I can take." Sir William Osler, the respected Canadian physician, perhaps best expressed what many doctors must feel. "When I see an arthritic patient walk in the front door of my office," he said, "I want to walk out the back door."

Most general practitioners know that there is little their conventional medicine can do to prevent or cure arthritis. The evidence of the efficacy of alternate therapies, however, is scientifically documented for anyone to see. If those practitioners would only turn to a more wholistic approach, they might not feel so helpless.

In Europe, herbs and cleansing diets have always been an important part of the medical cupboard – and are not considered quackery. There, an older, perhaps wiser, civilization would never think to scoff at any natural remedy that brings relief. Scientific interest in devil's claw root was sparked by the evidence of so many cured arthritics in England and Germany. There are hundreds of case histories already confirming the positive health benefits of the African desert root. And that herb is only one of a panoply of natural therapies.

It used to be that here in North America the wholistic approach – herbs, diet, vitamins, stress reduction, exercise – was found guilty even before it was tried. In future, orthodox medicine may have a hard time defending its vigorous rejection of what has helped so many people. A 1993 study done in Boston and reported in the *New England Journal of Medicine* finds that modern health seekers go more often to a wholistic health centre than they visit their regular doctor.

8

Non-Toxicity and Efficacy of Devil's Claw 410

Non-Toxicity Proven

A recent study by the Canadian Bureau of Drug Research showed again that devil's claw has no known toxicity.

A herbal remedy manufacturing and distributing company had recognized an urgent need when it offered devil's claw to Canadians suffering from arthritic pains and the discomforts of arthrosis. After becoming convinced of the efficacy of devil's claw, the company decided to import the herbal remedy to Canada. Demand for the devil's claw herb quickly rose, a sure sign that self-administered devil's claw therapy was working well. Was it working too well for the pharmaceutical giants selling various drugs for the treatment of arthritis?

In 1982 The Health Protection Branch (HPB) of Canada's Department of Health and Welfare asked the distributor for detailed information on devil's claw root and for samples. The HPB, it turned out, wanted to undertake a controlled efficacy and toxicity study of devil's claw, as apparently there was increasing "public" concern about the safety of devil's claw.

Understandably keen on learning the details of the study – a controlled, double-blind, comparative study done with mice and rats – the distributor contacted the HPB and was told that the tests performed showed devil's claw to be non-toxic.

However, the study did not find devil's claw significantly effective in reducing formaldehyde induced swellings, or edema.

It suggests that devil's claw does not work on artificially induced edema, except as a temporary analgesic, which is contrary to the results of previous studies cited. In any event, it does not negate the remarkable recovery experienced by thousands of people suffering from real arthritis caused not by formaldehyde injection, but by a number of other factors, which are unknown.

Efficacy of Devil's Claw Products

The Canadian government study does reemphasize that it is important to use only devil's claw 410 products made solely from the secondary root of devil's claw. This root contains the largest amount of active substances. Although devil's claw tea is very potent, it was found that due to its bitter taste, it is not taken as regularly as is necessary to obtain the full benefit of a treatment cycle. Fortunately, devil's claw is also available in tablet form. However, you should make sure that you buy only a product made from the extract of the original secondary storage root of the devil's claw plant. This extract should be of a concentration of 2:1, that is, 100 mg of the medicinal extract should be made from at least 200 mg of the original storage root. All studies mentioned in this book, including the new study, have been carried out with a tablet that contains at least 410 mg of the extract from 820 mg of the devil's claw root.

There are tablets on the market that consist only of

pressed herb powder. Also, there are capsules filled with the raw powder. Users should be warned against the purchase of such products as the original root powder is frequently found to be highly impure and may even contain harmful contaminants or bacteria. In the 410 extract tablet any possible contamination is completely eliminated by the extraction procedure, and in the preparation of the tea, any bacteria would be killed by contact with the boiling water.

In summary, to ensure a pure product you should insist on extract tablets that contain at least 410 mg of the devil's claw root extract which has been processed properly. The recommended dosage is 1230 mg extract, that is, three tablets of devil's claw root 410 daily; this corresponds to at least 2460 mg of pressed powder tablets.

Endnotes

1 Airola, Paavo, PhD, *How to Get Well*, Health Plus Publisher, Phoenix, AZ, p. 18, 1974.

2 Geist, Harold, PhD, *Psychological Aspects of Rheumatoid Arthritis*, Charles C. Thomas, Springfield, IL, pp. 4, 14, 19 1966.

3 Fredericks, Carlton, PhD, *Food Facts & Fallacies*, N.Y., pp. 208-9, 1974.

4 Davis, Adelle, *Let's Get Well*, N.Y., pp. 123-4, 1965

5 Selye, Hans, MD, *The Stress of Life*, Harper & Row, New York, NY, p. 54, 1976.

6 Ibid p. 165

7 There is a higher incidence among women.

8 Geist, loc cit. p. 4

9 Wade, Carlson, *Fact Book on Arthritis*, Nutrition and Natural Therapy, New Canaan, Connecticut, p.23, 1976

10 Schmidt, Siegmund, Zeitschrift für Naturheilkunde 22, 48, 1970.

11 Alive Books has on file many letters from readers and satisfied users. I cannot include all of these testimonials in this book, however, you may write to Alive Books to obtain copies of additional testimonials.

12 Zorn, Berhard, *Zeischrift für Rheumaforschung*, journal, 17,3/4,135,1958

13 Schmidt, loc cit.

14 *Therapiewoche*, 72,1072,1972.

15 *Deutsche Apotheker Zeitung*, 102, 1274, 1962.

16 The Arthritis Foundation, *The Truth about Aspirin for Arthritis*, NY, 1970.

17 Jayson, Malcolm & Allan St. J. Dixon, *Rheumatism & Arthritis*, London, p. 110. 1974.

18 *Medical World News*, April, 1974

19 Schmidt, Siegmund, *Die geistige Erde*, Origo-Verlag, Zurich, Switzerland, 1960.

20 Hoppe, H., *Erfahrungsheilkunde*, journal, pp. 7, 230, 1974.

21 The author refers to Namibians as South West Africans citizens of the former German colony of South West Africa, now Namibia.

22 Vogel, *Gesundheitsnachrichten*, July 1973 issue

23 von Korvin-Krasinski, *Die geistige Erde*, 1960.

24 *Inflammation... Investigation*, Toronto

25 Williams, Roger, *Nutrition Against Disease*, p. 122, 1971.

26 *Bestways Magazine*, pp. 4, 4, 64, 1977.

27 Dong, Collin H., *New Hope for the Arthritic*, Thomas Y. Crowell, N.Y.

28 Williams, loc cit. p. 123.

29 Treating of the causes of disease (in medicine).

30 Elwood, Cathryn, *Feel like a Million*, p. 228, 1973.

31 Davis, loc cit. p. 126.

32 Fredericks, loc cit. pp 210

33 *Journal of Orthomolecular Psychiatry*, pp. 6, 2, 114, 1977.

34 Fredericks, loc cit. pp212

35 I strongly recommend reading the two excellent books on the subject by Klaus Kaufmann: *Silica – The Forgotten Nutrient*, 1990, Alive Books, on vegetal silica from spring horsetail, and *Silica – The Amazing Gel*, 1993, Alive Books, on mineral silica from quartz crystals.

36 Haas, Elson M., MD, *Staying Healthy with Nutrition*, Celestial Arts, Berkeley, CA, pp 43-44., 1992.

37 Ibid, pp 48-49.

38 Ibid, pp. 258-260

39 Any salt of uric acid.

40 Hay, Howard,*Rheumatism & Arthritis*, Science of Life Books, Melbourne, p. 59. 1973.

41 Ibid

42 Sobel, Dava & Klein, Arthur C., *Arthritis: What Works*, St. Martin's Press, NY. 1989.

43 Dr. Hafström, Ingiäld, *Arthritis and Rheumatism* (as reported on p. 220 of *Arthritis: What Works* by Dava Sobel & Arthur C. Klein). 1988.

44 Haas, loc cit. pp 104-105, 108-109, 117-118

45 Ibid, p. 128

46 Williams, loc cit. pp. 124, 129.

47 Wade, loc cit. p. 59.

48 Howland, Donald, MD, *Arthritis*, SHG-Alive Books, Burnaby, BC.

49 Wade, loc cit. p. 67.

50 In the mid 1980s the Austrians developed a handy magnetic field neutralizer called ELMAG. This product and supporting literature for pain control is available through Teldon of Canada Ltd., 7528 Lambeth Drive, Burnaby, BC V5E 1Z4 or by telephoning (604) 436-0545.

Bibliography

Airola, Paavo. *How To Get Well*. Phoenix, AZ. Health Plus Publishers. 1974.
There Is a Cure for Arthritis. West Nyack, NY. Parker Publishing Co.
1968.

Alexander, Dan Dale. *Arthritis and Common Sense*. enlarged edition, West
Hartford, CT. Witkower Press. 1975.

The Arthritis Foundation, *The Truth about Aspirin for Arthritis*, NY, 1970.

Davis, Adelle. *Let's Get Well*. NY. Harcourt, Brace & World. 1965.

Dong, Collin H., *New Hope for the Arthritic*, Thomas Y. Crowell, NY.

Elwood, Cathryn. *Feel Like a Million*. NY. Devin-Adair. 1956.

Fredericks, Carlton and Herbert Bailey. *Food Facts & Fallacies*. NY. Arc.
1972.

Geist, Harold, PhD, *Psychological Aspects of Rheumatoid Arthritis*, Charles C.
Thomas, Springfield, IL, pp. 4, 14, 19 1966.

Dr. Hafström, Ingiäld , *Arthritis and Rheumatism* (as reported on p. 220 of
Arthritis; What Works by Dava Sobel & Arthur C. Klein). 1988.

Hoppe, H., *Erfahrungsheilkunde*, journal, pp. 7, 230, 1974

Howland, Donald, MD. *Arthritis*. SHG. Burnaby, BC. Alive Books

Jayson, Malcolm & Allan St. J. Dixon, *Rheumatism & Arthritis*, London, p.
110. 1974.

Kaufmann, Klaus, *The Joy of Juice Fasting*. Burnaby, BC. Alive Books. 1990.
Silica – The Forgotten Nutrient. Burnaby, BC. Alive Books. 1990.
Silica – The Amazing Gel. Burnaby, BC. Alive Books. 1993.

Mowrey, Daniel B., PhD. *The Scientific Validation of Herbal Medicine*.
Cormorant Books. 1986.

Science of Life Editorial Committee. *Rheumatism & Arthritis*. Melbourne.
Science of Life Books Pty. Ltd. 1944.

Schmidt, Siegmund, *Die geistige Erde*, Origo-Verlag, Zurich, Switzerland,
1960.
Zeitschrift für Naturheilkunde 22, 48, 1970.

Selye, Hans. *Stress Without Distress*. Philadelphia, PA. Lippincott. 1974
The Stress of Life. rev. ed. NY. McGraw-Hill. 1976.

Sobel, Dava & Klein, Arthur C. , *Arthritis: What Works*, St. Martin's Press,
NY. 1989.

Wade, Carlson. *Fact/Book on Arthritis, Nutrition and Natural Therapy*. New
Canaan, CT. Keats Publishing. 1976.

Williams, Roger J. *Nutrition Against Disease*. NY. Pitman. 1971.

Zorn, Berhard, *Zeischrift für Rheumaforschung* 17,3/4,135,1958

Index

A

acid, 6, 17, 32, 35, 41, 53-54, 56, 58-61,
    66-67, 83
acid-forming, 61, 67
acidophilus, 83
ACTH, 8, 54
adaptogen, xi
adrenal, 7-9, 36-37, 51-53, 66, 78
alfalfa, 43, 52, 56, 61, 66
allergy, 3-4, 56-57
allergy testing, 57
anemia, 18, 19
ankylosing spondylitis, 17
anti-stressor, 52
arm circles, 75
arm swing, 75
arsenic, 64
arterio, 20, 70, 81
arteriosclerosis, 28, 50, 81
ASA, 35
aspirin, 25, 35-36, 42, 53, 79, 85
autoimmunity, 4, 38

B

B complex, 14, 27, 33, 51, 53-54, 56,
    82-83
B12, 67, 83
B3, 53, 58, 66
B5, 66
B6, 58
bacillus, 5
bacteria, 8, 52, 66, 89
beryllium, 65
betacarotene, 59, 83
blood urea, 32
bony spurs, 10, 55
bromelain, 62
burdock, 43
bursitis, 18, 66

C

cadmium, 64

caffeine, 82
calcium, 10-11, 55-56, 67, 76, 83
cancer, 38, 50, 52, 81
capsule, 15, 89
cartilage, 3, 5, 10-11, 15-16, 52
cayenne, 43, 83
celery seed, 43
chaparral, 43
chloroquine, 38
cholesterol, 32, 40, 60, 73
choline, 54, 83
chondroitin sulphates, 83
chromium, 83
cod liver oil, 56, 59-60
coenzyme Q10, 83
collagen, 3, 14, 17, 33, 52, 67
comparative study, 88
connective tissue, 3, 14, 17-18, 33, 52,
    55, 66
copper, 56, 64, 83
corticosteroid, 32, 37
cortisone, 6, 8-10, 36-37, 42, 52-53, 67
crystallization, 59
cysteine, 58
cystine, 59

D

decosahexaenoic acid, 60
detoxification, 63, 65
Devil's Claw 410 Tablets, 23, 25, 88-89
DHA, 60
diabetes, 28, 40, 50
diagnostic, 57
diuretic, 32-33, 40
DL-phenylalanine, 58
dosage, 30, 32, 36, 83, 89

E

EFA, 59
eicosapentaenoic acid, 60
EPA, 60
ergosterol, 76
essential fatty acid, 56

Other titles by Alive Books

Fats That Heal Fats That Kill
The complete guide to fats, oils, cholesterol and human health.
Udo Erasmus, 1993, 480 pp softcover

Healing with Herbal Juices
A practical guide to herbal juice therapy: nature's preventative medicine. Siegfried Gursche, 1993, 240 pp softcover

Silica – The Forgotten Nutrient
Healthy skin, shiny hair, strong bones, beautiful nails. A guide to the vital role of organic vegetal silica in nutrition, health, longevity and medicine. Klaus Kaufmann, 1993, 128 pp softcover

Silica – The Amazing Gel
An essential mineral for radiant health, recovery and rejuvenation.
Klaus Kaufmann, 1993, 176 pp softcover

The Joy of Juice Fasting
For health, cleansing and weight loss.
Klaus Kaufmann, 1990, 114 pp softcover

Making Sauerkraut and Pickled Vegetables at Home
The original lactic acid fermentation method.
Annelies Schoeneck, 1988, 80 pp softcover

How to Fight Cancer and Win
Scientific guidelines and documented facts for the successful treatment and prevention of cancer and related health problems.
William L. Fisher, 1988, 297 pp softcover

Cancer – There is Hope
Alternative treatments, testimonials of cures, the Essiac story and more. Byrun F. Tylor, 1993, 128 pp softcover

Allergies: Disease in Disguise
How to heal your allergic condition permanently and naturally.
Carolee Bateson-Koch DC ND, 1994, 224 pp softcover

All of these books are available at your local health food store or from
Alive Books, PO Box 80055, Burnaby, BC V5H 3X1